FOR Dummies™
BESTSELLING
BOOK SERIES

Living Longer

D0014010

Cheat Sheet

The Three Keys to Living Longer: Exercise, Diet, and Rest

Exercise

An inactive lifestyle can contribute to one or more of the following six health conditions:

- Cardiovascular vulnerability
- Musculoskeletal fragility
- Immunologic susceptibility
- Obesity
- Depression
- Premature aging

To combat the onset of those conditions, incorporate the following four types of exercise into your daily routine:

- Aerobics
- Strengthening
- Flexibility
- Balance

Diet

The path to a healthful eating regimen is not through pills and fads. The best way is the most basic: Follow the Food Pyramid!

Rest

Here are some tips to get a better night's sleep:

- **Avoid stimulants.** Stop taking items such as coffee, chocolate, tea, and nicotine. Your brain doesn't need chemical clamor as it winds down.

- **Mind the bladder.** Tend to your pet's and your own toilet needs before retiring. A full bladder is an alarm clock.

- **Avoid heavy exercise before retiring.** All the gears of the body and mind need to be in neutral for sleep to find a happy haven.

- **Don't eat a big meal just before bedtime.** A full belly means the body must attend to its needs and in so doing keeps the machinery going.

- **Don't nap.** A good night's sleep quota can be robbed by gratifying the rest need early in the day.

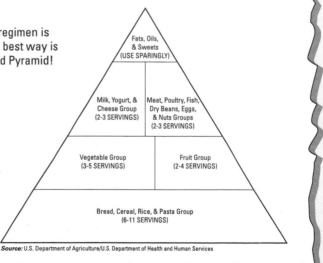

Fats, Oils, & Sweets (USE SPARINGLY)

Milk, Yogurt, & Cheese Group (2-3 SERVINGS)

Meat, Poultry, Fish, Dry Beans, Eggs, & Nuts Groups (2-3 SERVINGS)

Vegetable Group (3-5 SERVINGS)

Fruit Group (2-4 SERVINGS)

Bread, Cereal, Rice, & Pasta Group (6-11 SERVINGS)

Source: U.S. Department of Agriculture/U.S. Department of Health and Human Services

Drugs commonly used by older people

- **Blood thinners.** These drugs, such as coumadin, are used to keep the blood from clotting. Clotting is frequent in situations of prolonged bed rest or after surgery.

- **Anti-cancer drugs.** Because cancer is an overproduction of cells, the drugs designed for its treatment work by blocking cell division.

- **Anti-inflammatory medicines.** These compounds, including aspirin, are probably the most widely used class of medicine in older patients due to the high incidence of arthritis in an aging population.

- **Antibiotics.** These drugs are widely used to combat infection in patients of all ages and are far over-prescribed.

- **Cardiovascular drugs.** Hundreds of kinds of cardiovascular drugs address conditions from high blood pressure and high cholesterol to weak heart action and irregular heart beat.

- **Central nervous system medications**. Depression, hostility, and insomnia are common conditions in older populations.

- **Hormones.** For males, doctors prescribe testosterone in efforts to enhance flagging sexuality and vitality. For females, estrogen and progesterone have their value in offsetting cardiovascular problems, osteoporosis, and Alzheimer's disease.

You know it's an emergency when...

- There's a lack of breathing or pulse.
- The person is unconscious.
- You notice a major change in mental state (confusion, drowsiness, and so forth).
- There's active major bleeding.
- The person suffers from shortness of breath at rest.
- Someone experiences severe pain.
- A major injury is apparent.
- Ingestion of excessive medications or other toxic substances has taken place.
- There's an inability to urinate or have a bowel movement.

Normal Ranges for Bodily Functions

Pulse	45–80 per minute
Respiration	8–20 per minute
Temperature	97–99.5°F
Blood pressure	130/85–90/60 mmHg

Hungry Minds™

For Dummies®: Bestselling Book Series for Beginners

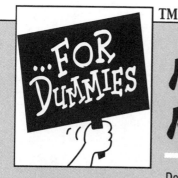 ™

References for the Rest of Us!®

BESTSELLING BOOK SERIES

Do you find that traditional reference books are overloaded with technical details and advice you'll never use? Do you postpone important life decisions because you just don't want to deal with them? Then our *For Dummies*® business and general reference book series is for you.

For Dummies business and general reference books are written for those frustrated and hard-working souls who know they aren't dumb, but find that the myriad of personal and business issues and the accompanying horror stories make them feel helpless. *For Dummies* books use a lighthearted approach, a down-to-earth style, and even cartoons and humorous icons to dispel fears and build confidence. Lighthearted but not lightweight, these books are perfect survival guides to solve your everyday personal and business problems.

> *"More than a publishing phenomenon, 'Dummies' is a sign of the times."*
>
> — The New York Times

> *"...you won't go wrong buying them."*
>
> — Walter Mossberg, Wall Street Journal, on For Dummies books

> *"A world of detailed and authoritative information is packed into them..."*
>
> — U.S. News and World Report

Already, millions of satisfied readers agree. They have made For Dummies the #1 introductory level computer book series and a best-selling business book series. They have written asking for more. So, if you're looking for the best and easiest way to learn about business and other general reference topics, look to For Dummies to give you a helping hand.

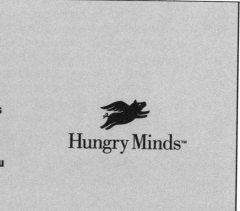

Hungry Minds™

1/01

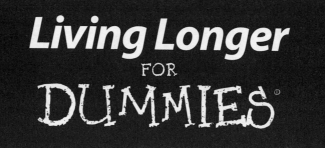

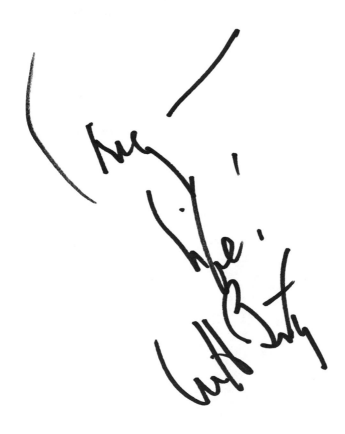

Living Longer

FOR

DUMMIES®

by Dr. Walter Bortz

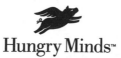

Hungry Minds™

HUNGRY MINDS, INC.

New York, NY ◆ Cleveland, OH ◆ Indianapolis, IN

Living Longer For Dummies®

Published by:
Hungry Minds, Inc.
909 Third Avenue
New York, NY 10022
www.hungryminds.com
www.dummies.com

Library of Congress Control Number: 00-112172

ISBN: 0-7645-5335-6

Printed in the United States of America

10 9 8 7 6 5 4 3 2 1

1B/QU/QU/QR/IN

Distributed in the United States by Hungry Minds, Inc.

Distributed by CDG Books Canada Inc. for Canada; by Transworld Publishers Limited in the United Kingdom; by IDG Norge Books for Norway; by IDG Sweden Books for Sweden; by IDG Books Australia Publishing Corporation Pty. Ltd. for Australia and New Zealand; by TransQuest Publishers Pte Ltd. for Singapore, Malaysia, Thailand, Indonesia, and Hong Kong; by Gotop Information Inc. for Taiwan; by ICG Muse, Inc. for Japan; by Intersoft for South Africa; by Eyrolles for France; by International Thomson Publishing for Germany, Austria and Switzerland; by Distribuidora Cuspide for Argentina; by LR International for Brazil; by Galileo Libros for Chile; by Ediciones ZETA S.C.R. Ltda. for Peru; by WS Computer Publishing Corporation, Inc., for the Philippines; by Contemporanea de Ediciones for Venezuela; by Express Computer Distributors for the Caribbean and West Indies; by Micronesia Media Distributor, Inc. for Micronesia; by Chips Computadoras S.A. de C.V. for Mexico; by Editorial Norma de Panama S.A. for Panama; by American Bookshops for Finland.

For general information on Hungry Minds' products and services please contact our Customer Care department; within the U.S. at 800-762-2974, outside the U.S. at 317-572-3993 or fax 317-572-4002.

For sales inquiries and resellers information, including discounts, premium and bulk quantity sales and foreign language translations please contact our Customer Care department at 800-434-3422, fax 317-572-4002 or write to Hungry Minds, Inc., Attn: Customer Care department, 10475 Crosspoint Boulevard, Indianapolis, IN 46256.

For information on licensing foreign or domestic rights, please contact our Sub-Rights Customer Care department at 650-653-7098.

For information on using Hungry Minds' products and services in the classroom or for ordering examination copies, please contact our Educational Sales department at 800-434-2086 or fax 317-572-4005.

Please contact our Public Relations department at 212-884-5163 for press review copies or 212-884-5000 for author interviews and other publicity information or fax 212-884-5400.

For authorization to photocopy items for corporate, personal, or educational use, please contact Copyright Clearance Center, 222 Rosewood Drive, Danvers, MA 01923, or fax 978-750-4470.

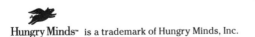

Hungry Minds™ is a trademark of Hungry Minds, Inc.

About the Author

Walter Bortz, M.D., is a specialist in internal medicine with the Palo Alto Medical Foundation in California and is a clinical associate professor of medicine at Stanford University. He was also the co-chairman of the American Medical Association's Task Force on Aging and the past president of the American Geriatrics Society.

Dr. Bortz has published over 100 scholarly papers in academic and medical journals as well as articles in *The New York Times, Washington Post, San Francisco Chronicle, Town & Country,* and *Runner's World.* His best-selling books include *We Live Too Short and Die Too Long* and *Dare To Be 100.* Dr. Bortz is also a lecturer and wellness advocate.

At 70 years of age, Dr. Bortz is an avid runner and has completed over 20 marathons, including Boston 2000, and he is the grandfather of nine.

Dedication

I am persuaded by whoever observed that a person's life achieves less significance by what he/she does than by that which that life causes to happen in others. I dedicate, therefore, this book to our grandchildren, Kellen, Taylor, Ryan, Don, Rosie, Tenly, Carson, Emily, and Eddie, and to your own, now and future. I hope their lives are the better by virtue of what we have learned and pass on.

Author's Acknowledgments

The sources of this book are many. First, there was Carol Mann, agent, who was there at the right time and has remained a steady advocate. Then, Julie Clark, super-transcriptionist, who took my often illegible yellow tablet scribbles and made them ink on white. Warm thanks. Then the Hungry Minds team, particularly Michael Cunningham, who translated my professorese to dummy-ease. Thank you. Family all ways and always. Patients, friends, colleagues, and many others, thanks.

Finally, I want to acknowledge books. Next to people, books are my most treasured asset. Books of all ages and content. My home study overflows with them. Aging invites warm comment from scientists, poets, economists, ethicists, politicians. Gardner, Finch, Friedan, Cousins, Cassell, Heilbrunn, Carter, Delaneys, Sagan, DeChardin, James, Evans, Erikson, Pauling, Gould, Hayflick, Carstensen, Tolstoi, and Sheehan mix freely on my shelves. Books nourish and inspire. I pray the electronic age does not cause their extinction. You can't cradle a computer. The computer can't be your good friend. Books are — thank you books.

Publisher's Acknowledgments

We're proud of this book; please send us your comments through our Online Registration Form located at www.hungryminds.com.

Some of the people who helped bring this book to market include the following:

Editorial

Project Editor: Linda Brandon

Acquisitions Editor: Michael Cunningham

Copy Editor: Corey Dalton

Acquisitions Coordinator: Stacy Klein

Technical Editor: Jean Macdonald, R.N.

Senior Permissions Editor:
Carmen Krikorian

Editorial Manager: Christine Beck

Editorial Assistant: Jennifer Young

Cover Photos: The International Stock©, Peter Iangone; Hi-Res in production

Production

Project Coordinator: Jennifer Bingham

Layout and Graphics: Kelly Hardesty, Jacque Schneider, Julie Trippetti, Jeremey Unger

Proofreaders: David Faust, Susan Moritz, Angel Perez, Nancy Price, York Production Services, Inc.

Indexer: York Production Services, Inc.

Special Help
Esmeralda St. Clair

General and Administrative

Hungry Minds, Inc.: John Kilcullen, CEO; Bill Barry, President and COO; John Ball, Executive VP, Operations & Administration; John Harris, CFO

Hungry Minds Consumer Reference Group

Business: Kathleen A. Welton, Vice President and Publisher; Kevin Thornton, Acquisitions Manager

Cooking/Gardening: Jennifer Feldman, Associate Vice President and Publisher

Education/Reference: Diane Graves Steele, Vice President and Publisher; Greg Tubach, Publishing Director

Lifestyles: Kathleen Nebenhaus, Vice President and Publisher; Tracy Boggier, Managing Editor

Pets: Dominique De Vito, Associate Vice President and Publisher; Tracy Boggier, Managing Editor

Travel: Michael Spring, Vice President and Publisher; Suzanne Jannetta, Editorial Director; Brice Gosnell, Managing Editor

Hungry Minds Consumer Editorial Services: Kathleen Nebenhaus, Vice President and Publisher; Kristin A. Cocks, Editorial Director; Cindy Kitchel, Editorial Director

Hungry Minds Consumer Production: Debbie Stailey, Production Director

◆

The publisher would like to give special thanks to Patrick J. McGovern, without whom this book would not have been possible.

◆

Contents at a Glance

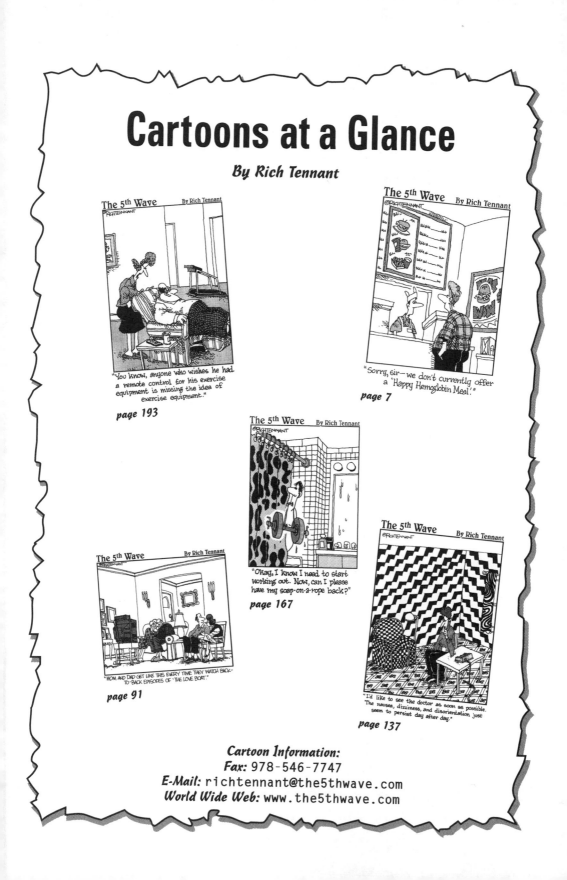

Table of Contents

Introduction

*W*riter Mae Sarton said, "As I age, I become more me." My hope is that this book may help you to become more "you" as you age. Becoming yourself is the ultimate human fulfillment story.

If you are lucky, you will grow old. The alternative is no fun at all. As George Burns observed, death "leaves you with too much free time on your hands." In this book, you will find that the issue of getting old is less about how long you will live, but how well you will age, and what your quality of life will be.

You can choose infinite paths to growing old. Some take the high road, some the low road. Most of us are somewhere in between. People who take the high road will live longer than those on the low road. My hope is to be able to inform and inspire you to take paths leading to the higher life.

When you live a long life, you get the opportunity to look back on acres of achievements accomplished and satisfactions gained. Achieving a good long life isn't easy. Going on that path takes effort and time. Many people don't want to make the effort to pursue the high road — it takes energy, engagement, and courage.

We are fortunate to be alive at this moment in history. We know more today about growing old than ever before. Until now, growing old was rare and random; a few people grew old, but not many. Nine of the thirteen children of Emperor Antoninus, A.D. 160, died in infancy. Only two of Mozart's nine children lived to adulthood. Those who made it to old age got there by chance. Now most of us should make it by design.

A football game is not over until the fourth quarter is finished. The race is not over until the last lap is run. A crossword puzzle isn't done until the last word is filled in. Dying before we have a chance to grow old means our life is not completed. We need to fulfill our design, which has been so tenderly and magnificently handed to us. We need to live into our old age.

I am a physician, so much of this book has a medical flavor, but I want you to know that aging is not a disease. Aging should not be medicalized. My career has been that of a geriatrician. I have learned largely from experience, because when I was a young doctor no formal training existed for geriatricians. Learning about the health problems of thousands of aging patients was on-the-job training.

I learned and I aged. What I learned from treating aging patients has been a wonderful curriculum for my own life. I learned that aging is all about choice. The older you become, the more you realize you are a byproduct of choices you made. I also learned how unimportant the doctor is in the whole business of growing older. Your ancestors contribute 20 percent to the extent of your life, your physician provides another 10 to 20 percent, and you determine the rest. Living longer is a choice, not fate. Living longer is active, not passive. You create your own destiny.

And while the body inevitably is involved in the process of aging, so too is the mind. The body is programmed to follow a slow, declining trajectory of form and function. The mind, on the other hand, has the opportunity to use time to its advantage. Flow, wisdom, creativity, emotional stability, tolerance, and perspective are all gained by living long. Like wrinkles on the face and knobs on the knees, emotional maturation is an integral part of the aging experience. If you live life well, your emotional maturity will validate and exalt the experience. At the end of your life, you must be able to say, "Yes, I lived." Too many people are born and then die with little in between. As literary figure and humanitarian Norman Cousins cautioned, "Too many people worry about whether there is life after death. Worry instead about whether there is life before."

I have been lucky to be taught by some great minds. My main teachers have been my patients. Although the pretense was that I was taking care of them as they aged, the reality was that they were teaching me. I have also been taught by some authors, whose writings I have read extensively. These writers extend from the hard sciences of physics and chemistry, through the middle ground of medical science, to the softer sciences of psychology, sociology, and anthropology. I have learned from lab scientists, ethicists, economists, masseuses, athletes, and artists. I have tried to learn about aging wherever and whenever the opportunity presented itself. Being a grandfather nine times has given me yet another perspective from which to learn what a full life may become.

Aging is a rich domain to explore. Most of the things we are discovering are good news: Growing older need not be a grim, forbidding picture. The negative imagery of aging arises because aging has been inadvertently mixed in with other misadventures that sometimes happen to older people, such as becoming frail. Becoming frail, however, is not actually part of the aging process. You can't cure aging, but you can prevent many negative aspects wrongly linked to growing old.

About This Book

There are many good books on aging out there. Some are almost mathematical, some are almost poetic. I hope that this book is part science and part art. I believe that science and art intersect and become mutually supportive. The process of aging cannot be reduced either to science or philosophy alone. I like to think of *Living Longer For Dummies* as a whole-life catalog with something for everyone. Men and women, young and old, are all involved in the aging process — and it's never too early or too late to learn.

I could not have written this book when I was 30, 40, 50, or even 60. There was still too much tread on my tires to know what the road really feels like. At 70, I started to be able to feel the road, and I hope you will too, someday.

The book is a reference book, and each part can be read separately. You can start at the back or the middle, and as someone once said, "Life has to be lived forwards, but it must be understood backwards." Certain themes emerge. I hope I have avoided dogmatism, but I do think some points are really important, and I have repeated and over-stated them for a reason. This book explores hard and important parts of life. I never intend to trivialize the tough issues, but neither do I wish to get overly serious if it's not necessary. I am sure that some of the ideas, with time, will be proven wrong, just as any survey book written even a decade ago will contain material that a brighter, stronger lens will reveal as mistakes.

The book is wider than it is deep. In the effort to portray a whole panorama of how best to live longer, I have included virtually all the topics that affect that process. There is so much of value to learn about the process of maturing, modern and otherwise, that no single book can provide more than a mention with notes. I encourage you to join me in learning about what seems to matter most. Look at this book as a first step toward the rest of your life. *Living Longer For Dummies* is the appetizer that prepares you for the rest of the meal.

The information in this reference is not intended to substitute for expert medical advice or treatment; it is designed to help you make informed choices. Because each individual is unique, a physician must diagnose conditions and supervise treatments for each individual health problem. If an individual is under a doctor's care and receives advice contrary to information provided in this reference, the doctor's advice should be followed, as it is based on the unique characteristics of that individual.

Foolish Assumptions

If you're reading this book about living longer, I'm assuming that you are what behaviorists call a "contemplator." A contemplator is ready to move but not yet committed to action. The contemplator is ready to consider. Maybe you are a *...For Dummies* fan who has just been waiting for a book on living longer. Maybe you are looking for ways to live a longer, healthier life and have just been waiting for the *...For Dummies* translation. But by whatever route you got here, welcome. I hope your reading will be worth the effort. If not, don't burn this book, just give it to some other contemplator who is ready to take action!

How This Book Is Organized

This whole-life catalog for living longer is divided into 13 chapters, five Parts of Ten, and two appendixes. The chapters are grouped into four parts with broad correspondence within the parts. Cross-referencing is provided between the chapters where related information is included.

Part I: The Mental and Physical Aspects to Living Longer

Yes, Virginia, there is a Santa Claus, and he is growing older. But you won't notice because he has already read this book. He has learned aging happens to everyone, and that his preconceived notions about aging were wrong. Chapter 1 explains what aging is and isn't. This is new, hot stuff, because until now almost all the labels about aging were wrong. Chapter 2 helps you understand the whole healthcare system. Chapters 3 through 5 cover the critical points to living longer, the points that I'll try to pound into your brain: exercising, eating right, and getting enough rest. Chapter 6 rounds out this part with information on alternative medicine and exercise techniques. This is crucial knowledge to making a life plan. Don't miss out.

Part II: The Psychological Aspects to Living Longer

Keeping your brain healthy is just as important as keeping your body healthy as you strive to live longer. Check out Chapter 7 for ways to maintain your brainpower. One way to keep your brain busy is to continue working or keeping up with activities of interest after you retire — and Chapter 8 shows you the way. Also don't forget about the importance of sex. Sex and aging has gotten a bad rap in the past, but Chapter 9 disproves some of the myths about sex and the aging person and gives you tips on how to continue a healthy sexual lifestyle well into your later years. The last chapter in this part, Chapter 10, gives pointers on how to ease your mind as far as where you will spend your last years.

Part III: Handling a Health Crisis

The thought of having to go to the emergency room is a scary one, but it is a fear that can be eased if you've thought through the process. Part III puts you on the path to demystifying the emergency experience. Chapter 11 starts you off by explaining your role in an emergency. How can you better prepare yourself? What should you expect after you're in the emergency room? This chapter answers those questions. Chapter 12 puts you in charge of your hospital experience by showing you some things you can do to take control of the type of experience you will have after you're in the hospital. Finally, Chapter 13 discusses surgery and the aging person.

Part IV: The Part of Tens

A favorite among ...*For Dummies* fans, The Part of Tens contains the choicest points of the book. Chapter 14 hands you the keys — ten of 'em! — to a healthy life. Chapter 15 doesn't let you just sit around, it shows you ten reasons to get moving instead. Chapter 16 gives you ten diet tips to fight the aging process while Chapter 17 tackles the ten ways to keep your mind in use. Finishing up, Chapter 18 takes on the important task of giving you ten guidelines to follow for taking medication safely.

Appendixes

The Appendix is a place for me to supply you with some nuts-and-bolts information. Think of it as the place to turn when you need information fast. Appendix A discusses taking medication with a list on the most common drugs used by older people that you may need to refer to in the coming years. Appendix B offers some handy tables on the most common conditions older people suffer from and the treatments that can be used.

Icons Used in This Book

Look for this icon to indicate that a story to help put the topic in perspective is approaching.

Be prepared to gain some of my precious insights — freely given, of course!

Here's where I offer some take-home messages to last a lifetime.

 These small hints will help make taking the bumps a bit easier.

 This icon cautions you that potential hazards lie ahead.

Where to Go from Here

The introduction is the end of the beginning and a broad template of the rest of the book. I hope that as you read you may pick up ideas and information that will allow you to become more you.

Part I

The Mental and Physical Aspects of Living Longer

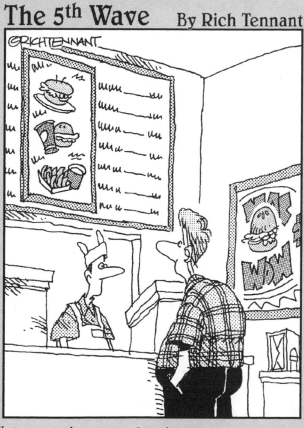

The 5th Wave   By Rich Tennant

"Sorry, sir—we don't currently offer a 'Happy Hemoglobin Meal.'"

In this part . . .

Aging is not something that you suffer through. It is a natural progression of life that brings lots of opportunities to try new things and to contribute what you've learned along the way. This part is set up to give you a good understanding of what aging is all about and how to live a long and healthy life.

Chapters 1 and 2 start you off right with overviews of the aging process and today's healthcare system. Get ready to get your body in shape as you read through Chapters 3, 4, and 5. These are the chapters where I establish the recurring themes of the book: eat right, exercise, and get enough rest. Finally, Chapter 6 will help to demystify the aspects of alternative medicines and exercise techniques.

Chapter 1

What in the World Is Aging Anyway?

● ●

In This Chapter

▶ Living a good long life

▶ Aiming for 100 and beyond

▶ Fulfilling life's promise — three sturdy strategies

▶ Understanding the three components to good health

● ●

*H*ow long is a good long life? 65 years? 78? 110? Most people haven't thought about the answer at all. Without any scientific guidelines, they were simply preoccupied with getting through each day. The few people who have thought about it were wrong.

One of the greatest gifts to present-day humankind is a firm prediction of how long we can live. Previous predictions fell far short of the reality of the human 120-year life span. The scientific establishment has newly identified one hundred twenty years as the true potential of the human organism. One hundred and twenty years is the human life span, which hasn't changed in hundreds of thousands of years, and is further unlikely to change any time soon. The life expectancy, on the other hand, has changed dramatically. The term *life expectancy* represents the actuality of how long we have lived, unlike *life span,* which represents our potential. Until now, everyone has died too soon, but we are getting better at living longer.

We have succeeded in getting rid of many of the scourges that have prematurely snuffed the lives of billions of our ancestors. Take starvation, for example. Most of our earliest relatives died because they didn't get enough to eat, unlike contemporary periods when a nutritional problem in developing countries is having too much food. After the Agricultural Revolution of 10,000 years ago, infections — smallpox, tuberculosis, plague, malaria, AIDS, and so forth — took over as the number one demon. The list of killer diseases is long and impressive with millions of casualties to claim. These premier killers are currently coming under control, however, revealing a whole new set of chronic degenerative conditions — such as heart disease, cancer, stroke, and diabetes — that conspire to barricade us from our 120-year life span opportunity. Fortunately, our knowledge of the new risks that we encounter with these conditions is also rapidly expanding, yielding the promise of fulfillment of the human life span potential for the first time in history.

Being "Old" Is New

Today, so many people live past age 65, you can say we're experiencing a worldwide epidemic of aging. The average age for life expectancy in the year 2000 is 78. In comparison, life expectancy was only 45 back in 1900, but it is predicted to increase to a whopping 100 by the year 3000! By that time, our society will have likely rubbed out the few gene-caused illnesses, eradicated infections and malignancies, and reconciled with the bad maintenance conditions (smoking comes to mind) that predominate today.

When is old? Two hundred years ago, anyone over 35 was old. Sixty years ago, I recall my 70-year-old grandparents as being "very old." Now, with the actual life span revealed to us, we know that "old" doesn't start until the start of the last third of life, at your 80th birthday, and that is "young old." "Old old" doesn't begin until you are 100. Dare to be 100.

Today, almost everyone in the world is living longer. Sweden leads the world in percentage of population over 65 with 17.9 percent. The United States is way down the list with 12.6 percent of the U.S. population currently over 65. Two million people in the United States turn 65 each year. However, immigration numbers and fluctuating birthrates both highly influence these statistics. In comparison, experts expect China, a country with a much younger population than either Sweden or the United States, to have 330 million persons over the age of 65 by 2050.

The effects of risk factors, or life habits that negatively impact longevity, are also important. I know of a group of nuns in Minnesota that has a life expectancy of almost 90 thanks to their elimination of many risk factors! When we eliminate all risk factors, we have the chance to die of aging.

We can reach age 100-plus

George Burns quipped that one of the reasons he looked forward to being 100 was that very few people over 100 die — because very few people live past the age of 100, of course! George Burns did live to see 100, and many more people are doing so as well. With so many more people now reaching 100, Hallmark is printing 70,000 Happy 100th Birthday cards this year. Willard Scott would go hoarse announcing all those names on NBC's Today Show!

The number of centenarians (people age 100 and over) increases 8 percent per year in the United States, contrasted to the overall population growth of 1 percent. We have certifiable evidence that living a long life is quite possible. In my office, I have a copy of the birth certificate of Madame Jeanne Calment, a French woman who was born February 21, 1875 and died August 4, 1997 — that's a lifetime of 122 years, 225 days — the longest on record! The record may not hold much longer, however, as millions of others are daily closing in on Madame Calment. Currently, the *Guinness Book of World Records* reports that Eva Morris of Staffordshire, England, is the world's oldest person having been born on Dec. 18, 1885.

Although Madam Calment and others have lived past 100 years of age, the century mark represents a more realistic and practical goal for all. Bob Butler, first director of the National Institute on Aging, wrote "We have not found any biologic reason to prohibit us from living to 100." The centenarians, the most rapidly growing segment of the population, give evidence of this possibility and its defining features.

Life at 100

Centenarians are almost by definition "successful agers." What about them makes them seemingly invulnerable to things that kill off other people of the same age?

Centenarians do seem to share some characteristics (see Table 1-1). Stability and a sense of equanimity and order rank high among their skills. Lack of anxiety and a capacity to get along with others are common attributes. Few loners live to be 100 and the ability to adapt is key to living that long. Exercise and the love of music both seem to help to confer long life.

How Madame Jeanne Calment reached 122+

Physicians reported Madame Calment's health as being pretty robust for her whole life. She retained vigor and attractiveness until shortly before she died. During her long lifetime, she lived in only three homes, leaving the second, a second-floor walkup apartment with no elevator, for a rest home at age 110. She broke her hip at 100, the last year she still ran for exercise. In fact, Madame Calment credited her exercise program for her health. She exercised once or twice daily and rode her bike until the age of 115. Madame Calment occasionally smoked a cigarette or a cigarillo after meals, but she quit at age 117. She also gave up her port, which was a long-time companion, but she never surrendered her chocolate, a dear love.

Table 1-1	Characteristics of Centenarians
Orderly	
Industrious	
Mobile	
Nonsmoker	
Frugal	
Optimistic	
Patriotic	
Frisky	
Religious	
Curious	

Your goal should not be just to reach a certain age, but to age in a healthy way that leaves you capable of enjoying life. This is a prize we can all strive toward — and one the rest of this book can help you achieve.

Defining Aging

Seeking to define what aging is and isn't reveals much more of what it isn't than what it is. Much of the negative imagery of aging isn't deserved, because many, if not most, of the bad features that have masqueraded as aging are, in reality, due to other processes. Aging isn't disease. Aging isn't genes. Aging isn't bad maintenance. Aging is a natural progression of life, a fundamental reality; so, the more you learn about what aging is, the better prepared you'll be for the challenges it brings.

Shockingly, almost everything that people have believed about aging until recently is wrong. If most of what people consider to be aging isn't, then what exactly is aging? To establish this definition, you need to survey what the master physicist Mother Nature had in her handbag when she created the whole universe in the first place. I submit that she had only three items in there:

- ✔ Matter
- ✔ Energy
- ✔ Time

Free radical demons

"Better living through chemistry" is truer than the Dupont Company slogan intends. We are each a large chemical furnace with billions and billions of reactions going on in our cells every second. Unfortunately, all the gears aren't perfect. All the combustions of sugar into carbon dioxide, water, and energy create ash, trash, and metabolic debris. Doctors call the debris of the chemical reactions that constitute life the *free radicals.* These tiny oxygen atoms are chemically unstable and negatively impact the other chemistry going on around them — like dirt in the crankcase. As a result, damage occurs: The membranes around cells become less permeable; the elastic tissue, such as that in the back of your hand or in your face, loses tone and starts to sag; the DNA of your cell growth machine becomes damaged. A whole range of bad things happens when free radicals are free to damage. The free radical theory, first proposed by Denny Harmon of Nebraska University, is the unifying explanation for aging.

That's all that existed at the start, and that's all that exists now. Only the distribution of these items has changed. The definition of aging, then, is *the effect of energy on matter over time.* The effect of an energy flow on matter is basically *unidirectional* — it goes in only one direction. Time gives the direction, which is why the effect of energy on matter has been called *time's arrow.* Cycles exist within time's one direction, such as seasons, tides, day, night, and so on. However, all the cycles embed themselves in the directed arrow of time. Seasons bring new beginnings and pregnancies bring new life, but the insistent march of time still drives these processes.

Aging from the outside

What are some examples of the effect of energy on matter? Erosion by waves or rain or wind is one example. The way the color of your car hood or your house changes because of exposure to sunlight is another. A car ages much faster if you drive it 30,000 miles a year in dust or sleet rather than leaving it safely in the garage under wraps. In these examples of aging in the nonliving world, the energy of aging comes only from an external source.

Aging from the inside

For living creatures such as ourselves, not only do external sources disturb our matter such as sunlight causing premature skin wrinkling, but inside ones do so as well. The machinery of chemistry, called *metabolism,* drives life. Metabolism allows life by assembling billions and billions of chemical reactions in such a miraculous way that order arises out of chaos. In life's beauty, however, lies a flaw — aging. Aging is the price we pay for being alive, because the aliveness involves chemical reactions that, like your car and heater, generate trash — otherwise known as free radicals. This trash accumulates over time to yield what we call aging.

Wear, tear, and repair

So aging is simply wear and tear, from external and internal energy sources. The more energy impacting adversely on a canyon or a canary or a car, the quicker it ages. Shoes worn daily wear out seven times faster than shoes worn once a week.

Luckily, living creatures have an incredible capacity for self-repair. A Chevy can't repair its own dented fender, but the human body can repair a bruised backside. In fact, our capacity for repair is one of our most amazing abilities. We doctors would be in a terrible fix if bodies didn't heal themselves. Physicians take a lot of credit for things that the body does on its own. A doctor focuses on preventing or reversing situations that may keep the body's own repair capacity from functioning, such as infections or poor circulation, but medical effort, by itself, doesn't heal. Doctors simply assist self-healing.

One major aspect of our repair capacity is directed against the harm caused by the ash and debris that our metabolism generates. The wear and tear of living is the cause of aging, but the repair mechanism reverses only part, not all, of aging. The equation, then, for aging for a living creature is:

Wear + tear − repair = aging

Theoretically, if repairs were perfect, we would suffer no real loss of structure and function due to age. If a canyon wall could rebuild itself as fast as the water erodes it, no real change would occur. If our cells could undo the havoc caused by the imprecision of metabolism, we would register no real change. But so far, at least, this has proven to be an unmet challenge.

Reclassifying aging

A long list of infirmities involving all body parts and function — from hair and teeth to joints and sexuality — has characterized the ends of lives. These infirmities represent the stereotype of what aging is all about, and scanning the list is no fun.

How many of our infirmities must we accept, and how many can we change? How many of the infirmities are due to bad design? How many are due to aging? How many are due to disease? How many are due to bad maintenance? We are just now finding out the correct answers.

In 1982, I wrote an article in the *The Journal of the American Medical Association* entitled "Disuse and Aging." It included 111 references and borrowed heavily from literature that covered early space travel because most of the information about disuse — meaning characterizations of a sedentary lifestyle — was published there. According to this literature, the astro- and cosmonauts very rapidly developed negative changes commonly found in old people, which reversed themselves when they returned to earth. These changes obviously didn't occur because the astronauts became precociously old; they occurred because these space travelers broke free from the physical demands imposed on them by the gravitational forces. As a result of the systematic survey of many body systems, I concluded that most of the negative changes found in old people were not due to age, but to disuse and bad maintenance. This distinction is critical because aging is on the "accept" list, whereas disuse and bad maintenance are on the "do something about it" list.

Don't believe everything you read on a death certificate

In my role as a geriatrician, I have presided over the deaths of thousands of patients. For the year 1994, I kept a record of my patients who died. After they died, I reviewed their functional states six months, one month, and one week before their deaths. I recorded this experience in an article entitled "The Trajectory of Dying" in the *Journal of the American Geriatric Society*. Ninety-seven patients under my care died that year. (The high number represents the terminal state of these people more than my ability as a physician, I beg you to believe!)

The truth is, I really didn't know why most of them died — for most I simply received a call from a nursing home nurse telling me that my patient had died. The nurse usually answered my inquiry into what had happened with, "Nothing. We simply found him/her dead." I then had to fill out the death certificate to attest to the cause of death. Most commonly I wrote, "Cardiac arrest secondary to generalized arteriosclerosis." Translated, this means "heart stoppage due to clogged pipes." But I really didn't know.

Nonetheless, this death goes on the record as heart disease, but it could have been a stroke, or a blood clot, or possibly frailty. But doctors cannot accept "frailty" on a death certificate because it isn't a codeable diagnosis. In the old days, physicians could write simply "natural causes," but no longer. Doctors could never use "old age" as a diagnosis — probably correctly so, because very few people have ever lived long enough to die from old age. A survey of death certificates in Connecticut concluded that more than half was certifiably wrong. Renowned gerontologist Leonard Haflick wrote, "Few people over the age of 65 die from what is written on his or her death certificate. The real problem was not a particular illness, but whatever changes within the body that made it vulnerable to the illness."

My efforts to reclassify "aging" changes into their proper categories gained much momentum with the 1987 publication of Jack Rowe and Bob Kahn's article "Human Aging – Usual and Successful" in the journal, *Science*. This single article became the most influential one in the history of geriatric medicine because of the wonderful focus it provided for the Serenity Prayer precepts. (The Serenity Prayer reads, "God grant me the serenity to accept the things I cannot change, courage to change the things I can, and wisdom to know the difference.") Jack and Bob observed that whereas the great majority of older people conform to the "usual" model of aging with its attendant list of infirmities, others exist in the same age group, who somehow escape the demerits of the larger group. Their article emphasized that much of the stereotyping of aging simply doesn't hold true.

This relabeling of aging represents a huge conceptual shift, from the pessimistic, passive, accepting philosophic framework to an optimistic, action-oriented proposition. Such an interventionist effort is directed not only at lengthening life, but also at improving the quality of the added years as well.

Behaving responsibly about your health

One choice you must make for yourself is whether or not to behave responsibly about your health. You can choose to smoke, or you can remain smoke-free. You can choose to exercise, or you can sit on the couch. You can choose to eat potato chips and candy bars, or you can eat vegetables.

We must accept our starting place and our ending place in life, but we can change everything in-between. Humans are agents of change and, so, must take on the responsibility of healthy aging.

Three Sturdy Strategies to Help You Live Longer

Armed with the knowledge that you can live a very long life while maintaining your quality of life, what do you do now?

In my view, people are living longer because they know a lot more. The new knowledge base is increasingly available to all. I predict that the global advance in knowledge will do more to increase longevity than trains full of heart surgeons and new drugs. The following sections present you with even more knowledge and delineate three strategies for living longer.

Believing that you will live a long life

Aging truly is a self-fulfilling prophecy. How long you live is a direct result of your expectations. If you think you're going to be dead at 60, or 70, or 80, then that is likely to be the case. Or perhaps you think, "Well, maybe I won't be dead by then, but I will probably be in a forlorn nursing home with a plastic tube in my nose, endlessly contemplating ceiling tiles." Again, I believe that if you say you will end your days in a nursing home, you probably will.

Each day you behave in such a way as to guarantee the accuracy of your own prediction. Now, pretend you believe, "I'm going to live to be 100 because that is what I am programmed for." If you can stop pretending and truly believe that statement, then it is likely to come true. But, your behavior must support your prediction — and this book shows you just how you can do that!

To celebrate your 100th birthday means making a lot of right decisions and choices. Some people may live to be 100 by accident, most will make it by conscious choice. You are much more likely to arrive at your destination if you know where you are headed.

There is an increasingly large body of scientific proof of how attitude — good and bad — directly affects health outcomes. The mind and the body are no longer separate. You cannot make 100 without a healthy partnership between the two.

Believe in 100. Reaching 100 is your birthright, so not living to 100 is a discredit to your natural design.

Taking control of your life

To seize control of your destiny you must first recognize that *you* are responsible for living a long life. Neither your ancestors, your doctor, your family, your company, your pastor, nor the Social Security Administration is going to get you to a grand old age. You and you alone can get you there. You are in charge, not only of how long you will live, but, more importantly, of how well you will live. You can't delegate the task. In this more than anything, your destiny is what you make it. Of course, helpers exist along the way. No one is smart or strong enough to go it alone, but after all is said and done, you craft your own future.

Knowing it's never too late

No matter how old you are or what shape you're in, you can take steps to help reverse the process of aging that has already occurred and to slow your rate of aging in the future.

Lamenting, "If only I had started sooner," or "If only I had known about this," doesn't work. "If onlys" get you nowhere. The human organism's capacity to renew is vast, and the renewal capacity exists until the moment your toes curl up. Bones mend, and scrapes and scratches heal, even in centenarians. Using age as an excuse for being less than your best is just plain wrong.

Occasionally, a patient will visit my office in a wheelchair, and I eagerly inquire about why this mode of travel. "I'm 80!" comes the reply. I respond, "What's that got to do with anything? I expect you to walk in here on your next visit."

So remember what I call the *triple prescription* – three items that are the keys to living a long, healthy life:

- ✔ Believe that you will live a long life.
- ✔ Take control of your life.
- ✔ Understand it's never too late.

More and more people are getting this message. Don't get left out.

Understanding the Three Components of Health

Although thinking positively is an important part to living a longer and healthier life, it's only part of the challenge. To figure out what makes up health, pretend you are an athletic trainer and you're looking for the healthiest person on earth to be your client. How would you determine the criteria for healthiest person? My guess is the person would be a female, because women live longer. How old would she be? In her late 20s or early 30s, because her growth is done, and her physical capacities are at their highest. Assume the world's healthiest person asks you for advice on how to stay as healthy as she is at that moment. What is your advice for your new trainee? How do you help her sustain ultra-high performance?

I'll give you a hint: your advice should cover three main areas — exercise, diet, and rest. (You can find more specifics on these areas in Chapters 3, 4, and 5.) Within these three broad categories lie all the secrets of health. How can I validate this bold claim? Take away one of the three and see where you end up. For example, tell the woman to exercise and make sure to eat well, but to take no rests. Or, give her plenty of rest and exercise, but don't allow her to eat. Or allow her to eat and rest, but don't allow her to exercise. Any one of these three alternatives would lead to a profound loss of performance, and eventually poor health.

These three basics aren't glamorous. In fact, you've heard them all before, and really, the topics are pretty boring. Why should you exercise, or diet, or rest? The temptation to get a pill or a machine to do these things for you exists. As a last resort, many people figure they'll just pay the doctor to repair whatever bad results of their dereliction may come along. As an insider to the medical system, I caution you not to count on doctors to fix years of poor maintenance on your part. Again, prevention is key, even if it's not exciting or dramatic.

Physical exercise is the first of my two principal strategies for living a long and wonderful life. The second major strategy is social engagement, discussed later on in the book. Of the three components — exercise, diet and rest — I consider exercise to be the single most important one. I talk more about starting and maintaining a regular exercise program in Chapter 3.

We all need fuel to live. The kind of fuel you put into your body can determine how well your body runs, and how long it lasts. See Chapter 4 for more on diet.

Sleeping is not in vogue. In our busy society, being too occupied to sleep much is fashionable. How's a few hours' less of sleep per night going to hurt you, anyway? Quite a lot — and lack of sleep increases the speed of the aging process. See Chapter 5 for more on rest and relaxation.

Chapter 2

Getting Good Healthcare

● ●

In This Chapter

▶ Understanding the medical community

▶ Finding the best doctor for you

▶ Knowing your healthcare system

▶ Using alternative sources of healthcare support

● ●

*M*edicine has a proud and honored history as a profession. Not long ago, what the doctor said was "gospel," so to speak. People revered physicians for their knowledge and technical know-how, which was, and is, increasing by leaps and bounds. As medical advances continue, doctors are increasingly able to help in extending life, and more importantly, in improving the quality of life. The increased use of expensive technology and the aging of the population have led to efforts to control costs, managed care among them. Yet even with all the positive growth in the medical field, doctors still have room for improvement. With the advent of managed healthcare and the increased use of high-tech equipment, many patients are left with a long list of concerns and questions as to what's the best approach to get the right healthcare.

This chapter breaks down the complexities of today's medical system to help you understand how the system works and how to make it work for you. One of the most important decisions you'll need to make in life is choosing the best healthcare team. This chapter guides you through the process, showing you what questions to ask and what steps to take to make you a better, more informed patient.

Understanding the Medical System

Medicine has had three major historical eras. The first, the "don't challenge authority" era, lasted from Hippocrates' time until Ralph Nader. During that long interval, the doctor ruled. People accepted the physician's judgement, faulted as it was, as gospel. This one-sided approach lasted until the Vietnam War era when authoritarianism came under universal assault. Distrust of old ideas and institutions, as well as rejection of anything that smacked of "do as I tell you," flared. Patient rights were widely proclaimed, second and third opinions flourished, and medical information sources burgeoned. This "patient autonomy" era lasted less than two decades to be replaced by the third, and current, era of medical care. In this "administrative" era, decisions are no longer reached by the physician or by the patient, but by the insurance carrier. No one is happy about this sequence, but the current system is a predictable result of money. The run-up of the nation's healthcare costs was an extravagance that even the rich United States could not afford. Alarms were sounded that the United States couldn't compete in the international marketplace because its industries were saddled with healthcare costs that far exceeded those of any other country.

Coming to terms with the terms

Managed care and its most common form, Health Maintenance Organizations (HMOs) arose in an effort to hold down costs. The structure was brought about by a principle known as *prepaid medical care*. Prepaid care is an old Chinese way of paying for medical services. Pay the doctor on January 1 for the coming year, period. No more bills, regardless of what illness strikes. Prepaid care is in contrast to the standard fee for service model that works after the fact — get sick first, then pay. The prepaid model spawned the different organizational structures of managed care that follows:

- **HMO (Health Maintenance Organization):** Usually large numbers of health professionals of diverse types joined in one network, but at varied locations with a centralized general administration, with or without their own insurance program.

- **PPO (Preferred Provider Organization):** Aggregation of health professionals who through strength of numbers are joined to provide advantage in negotiating with health insurers.

- **IPA (Independent Practice Association):** Loosely, or nonaffiliated, health professionals with independent administrator and logistic practices who join together for increased access and leverage.

I grew up in the good old days when life was simple. A visit to the doctor involved only three people: a doctor, a nurse (who also served as the doctor's secretary and receptionist), and a patient. Fee-for-service medicine worked then. It was cheap. With the explosive growth in knowledge, however, came specialists in everything and machines for everything — and both of these cost big bucks. The old model died.

Logically, the doctors banded together in clinics, hospital groups, IPAs, PPOs, and assorted other arrangements, each supposedly designed to provide efficiency and restrained costs. It hasn't worked well as hoped — at least, not yet.

This new way of practicing medicine has lost the "caring" credential, which medicine has always carried with pride. The depersonalization, which seems so prevalent, discourages everyone involved. If you're not part of the solution, however, you're part of the problem. So, how can you be part of the solution? I offer two prime recommendations: be informed and communicate. With these two prescriptions already in your pocket, your medical encounters should be much improved.

Evaluating the impact of today's system

One helpful way to get a feel for how the medical system works is to survey the experience of 100 healthy middle-aged people. In one month, 75 of the 100 will experience some health matter, such as a splinter in the thumb, a cold, a headache, or depression. Of these 75, 25 will feel that the problem is intense enough to call their primary care physician. Of these 25, five will require further work-up, including a possible referral to a specialist. Of these five, one will need hospitalization and/or surgery.

Until now, the emphasis for these patients has been toward increasingly high-tech solutions to their problems. Now, in the new era of prepaid medical care, each patient visit is under review. Healthcare systems are seeking strategies that reduce, rather than increase, high-tech interventions.

The shift from high-tech solutions to other alternatives has been increasingly evident in the case of the dying person. Until recently, dying had become an in-hospital, high-tech act. This movement to the hospital was not precipitated by a well-reasoned process, but almost by default. Few people would choose to die in a hospital, given the choice, so why were they? A solution has come in the form of the hospice movement, a notable, new instrument that, when expanded and artfully employed, allows people to die at home. I don't want to die in an antiseptic chamber; I want to die in my own nest, made of my own materials, and peopled with persons whom I cherish and love. The Hospice movement can help make this possible.

I believe strongly in prepaid medical care, the old-fashioned Chinese way. In China, the patient pays a flat fee on January 1. That's it. If lightning strikes the patient, their once-a-year fee covers all costs. If nothing happens all year long, the doctors still provide basic maintenance. If the person's health profile improves because of better behavior practices, the insurance company reduces the premium for the next year. By risk-adjusting insurance premiums based on health behaviors, the medical system and the patient remain on the same page. Our health system should award *informed* health behavior and penalize those who knowingly undermine their health through poor behaviors.

Understanding Disease and Minimizing Your Risk

Understanding disease is even more important than understanding the healthcare system. After all, disease is what will cause you to enter the system in the first place. Becoming better informed about diseases that may potentially harm you, and knowing how to minimize your risk, can play an important role in choosing the healthcare provider that works best for you.

In the last century, doctors have matured in their understanding of disease. Physicians now identify disease for what it is — a condition often caused by an offending agent that, through its action, harms the patient. Such agents come in two principal varieties, infections and malignancies, both of which have changed over the course of centuries.

Recognizing the difference between infection and malignancies

The current spectrum of infection differs completely from the spectrum of infection a few years ago. Medical science has done a brilliant job of limiting the force of infectious disease. In the 1930s, my parents exiled me to the New Jersey seashore each summer because they feared that my hometown of Philadelphia's July or August weather would breed polio. Today, my children and grandchildren don't even know what polio is. The story is the same with smallpox and measles. I'm not sure I would even know how to diagnose a case of scarlet fever, a scourge a short while ago.

Malignancies, too, are yielding to medical science. The process is more difficult, but daily miracles occur in the cure of leukemia and lymphoma, which were uniformly fatal not long ago.

Infections result from some invading bug taking up residence in a person's body where it is not welcome. These can be viruses, bacteria, fungi, or worms. Malignancies, or cancer, on the other hand, are caused by some agent (cigarette smoke for example) upsetting the magnificently controlled genetic machinery responsible for cell growth and repair. Cancer occurs when the sequence of genes that monitor the orderly process of tissue regeneration becomes disorderly, and uncontrolled growth (cancer) results.

The treatments of infection and cancer have been the major business of medicine until now. The image of the physician as hero on the white horse slaying the disease dragon with a spear was established. But the shield is nobler than the spear. Prevention far exceeds cure in the greater scheme of things. And you the patient, fortunately, have a great deal to say about whether infections or malignancies will be your burdens to bear.

Prevention: More than half the cure

After you identify a disease as a real or potential problem, you can choose between two active strategies to change what you can change. The first strategy is cure, and the second is prevention. As I mentioned in the previous section, most of the medical research in the past century has gone toward the effort to cure, and successes abound. However, prevention holds the true glory.

Life would be better if preventive efforts closed the theater of disease, but the United States currently spends less than 2 percent of its national healthcare budget on prevention.

Someone observed that most doctors are so busy mopping up the spilled water that they neglect to turn off the spigot. Turning off the spigot is partially the physician's job, but it is mostly up to the public as a whole, which explains why I am so high on community health planning. In my view, everyone in your neighborhood needs to be more involved in health. Schools, churches, businesses, government, media — everyone. Health promotion and disease prevention needs to be the new focus of healthcare, instead of further increasing the power and expense of the curing function. The great majority of illnesses are preventable. So why don't people prevent them?

Health has three sturdy legs to stand upon, good exercise, good nutrition, and adequate rest. (See Chapters 3, 4, and 5 for more specifics!) All of these three are crucial, and all of them require regular and persistent personal involvement. The only good disease is the one that you prevent. Working with your doctor, you can develop this ideal health insurance policy.

Searching for Your Ideal Healthcare Team

In the "good old days," people maintained a trusted relationship with a doctor for many decades. Those days have departed. Today, both patients and physicians move around much more than they used to. Also, a new disruptive force exists in the doctor/patient relationship — the insurance plan. When employment changes, insurance changes, and often insurance — not the doctor/patient relationship — dictates the decision to find a new doctor.

Your first question when seeking a doctor used to be, "Who is a good doctor?" Now too often it is, "Which doctor is included in my insurance plan?" This added consideration complicates the process of selecting a new doctor.

The central questions you should answer in choosing a doctor include:

✔ **Is the doctor competent?** Ask about your physician's credentials: where and when did he/she attend medical school, did he/she complete postgraduate training, is he/she board certified, what medical associations does he/she belong to, what are his/her hospital affiliations? If you have a specific concern, address your potential doctor's expertise in that area. You always want to know whether or not your doctor has handled many cases like your own.

✔ **Does the doctor have good communication skills?** Authoritarianism is not a good posture for anyone, particularly a physician. Never do what your doctor says just because he or she says to do it. Knowing that your doctor shares your value system is critical. If you value preventative measures as your first line of defense against illness, as I hope you do, make sure that your physician is comfortable with this basic philosophy and is by your side as you follow through with this practice.

✔ **Are the doctor's services affordable?** Don't underestimate the cost issue as a deciding factor. Medical care is never cheap, and, for most people, it represents a major drain on the family resources. For this reason alone, you need a firm confidence in the appropriateness of your physician's charges. Be sure that your doctor is open to defending his or her reasoning for ordering certain tests and procedures — this way you'll be sure to understand your treatment and the importance of the services you're receiving.

✔ **How much time does the doctor have for you?** Please remember that the most important product you will buy from your doctor is time. Time is more significant than tests, procedures, or medicines, because time is what allows understanding. The fact that physicians' time is being more and more pinched, like everything else, is no secret. But your doctor's provision of time to you is where you will eventually find satisfaction or dissatisfaction with the care given to you. One technique to find out how a doctor utilizes time is to ask how many routine patients per hour does the doctor schedule. Anything more than four means your visit will be cramped.

✔ **How accessible is the doctor?** Early on, find out how long you should expect to wait for a routine appointment and how long scheduling a physical exam takes. A general rule is that routine appointments should not take more than 10 to 14 days to schedule — or one month for physical exams. If waits get longer, the doctor is too busy and either needs an associate or has too many patients. Don't let this happen to you.

✔ **How comfortable are you with the doctor?** Maybe liking your doctor is not a necessity, but it sure helps. Many medical encounters occur under difficult circumstances, and if you're asking for help in solving your problems, having a strong personal relationship with your physician makes a lot of sense. Your physician should be frank and fully disclosing about potential charges. A good physician has nothing to hide or be embarrassed about regarding finance or decisions on your healthcare.

Most people find a new doctor through word of mouth. Family and friends represent an information network and can be good indicators of what doctor will likely work out for you. If the word-of-mouth network doesn't pan out, call the county medical society or your local hospital for their list of suggestions. And if you wind up in trouble and find that you need a doctor, sometimes a resident physician in the emergency room can steer you in the right direction. They are usually well informed as to the best doctors in town. If you have a specific medical condition, such as Parkinson's disease, diabetes, or heart disease, the appropriate local service organization should give you names of competent physicians.

Decision-making ability is another key quality of a good physician. I have sometimes tried an informal inventory on the medical decisions I make on a daily basis: Why did I prescribe this medicine rather than that one and why for a certain number of days? Which tests did I order? Which phone calls did I answer directly versus delegating? When did I request hospitalization or consultation? When did I make a house call versus a phone call? At the end of the day, which last tasks get done and which are put off? The number of decisions I make each day clearly number into the hundreds. Consequently, just on a statistical basis alone, I will make a certain number of wrong decisions. Everyone makes mistakes, but physicians' mistakes are often more crucial. I know of no physician in my career that is indifferent to the likelihood of error somewhere, sometime. All patients should require from doctors is that we are up front about our decisions and move aggressively to minimize error. Your doctor should be straightforward with you about the medical decisions you make, and you should be able to participate so that you are making these decisions together.

From generalists to specialists

A primary care doctor is a general internist or a family practitioner. You need a primary care physician in your life more than you need a banker, hair colorist, barber, lawyer, or congressperson. This person helps you care for your most precious asset — your health.

Primary care means whole, continuous care for the entire person over time. No team of specialists and no computer program can assume the essential role of a primary care physician.

Being aware of the few "bad apples"

Like in every other profession, some physicians don't truly belong in medicine. Bad apples invade every crowd. Usually, these doctors operate on the fringes of medicine. They don't participate in or even belong to good hospitals or medical groups. Generally, a few direct questions can reveal whether a physician quacks or speaks the right language. Here are a few things to look out for:

✔ If the doctor prescribes three medicines per day — unless you are very sick.

✔ If you receive a new prescription on every office visit.

✔ If you receive a regular injection on every office visit.

✔ If you get unexplained costly services.

✔ If the doctor fails to do a physical examination.

✔ If the doctor repeatedly fails to respond to questions or requests.

✔ If you find poor ethical standards in reports or billing practices.

Fringe doctors are dangerous, and the records are full of misadventures encountered with unworthy physicians. All doctors make mistakes. Claiming the opposite is absurd. But a good doctor will acknowledge any mistakes and immediately take steps that ensure that the same mistakes don't happen again.

Medical specialists, sub-specialists, and sub-sub-specialists (I could go on, but you get the idea) are byproducts of the explosive increase in medical knowledge. The new information on every possible specialty that gushes from research centers is virtually impossible for a generalist to absorb. As a result, a good primary care physician ideally is a master of managing complexity and uncertainty, and so recognizes the extent of his/her competence and when to ask for consultation help.

Sometimes, but not always, a specialist may become your primary care doctor. Most specialists do not want this designation, but occasionally a cardiologist, endocrinologist, or rheumatologist may play the primary care role because of the need for frequent visits. But you should not assume that your specialist is playing this role for you. Ask directly whether the specialist will serve the nonspecialized role, including refilling prescriptions, undertaking physical exams, and being an all-around handy doc.

The idea of specialization is, of course, to apply a higher degree of skill to a tough problem. This aim is praiseworthy. The danger, however, is that specialization leads to fragmentation of the patient. When a team of physicians, each in charge of a part of you, administers care, the care becomes disjointed. Because a specialist's care tends to be episodic, responding largely to individual acute problems, a discontinuity of care may result. A specialist's ethic is to cure. The primary care doctor's role is to be there for the patient, both before and after the specialist's work is done. As I mention in Chapter 1, however, most medical conditions, particularly in old people, are not acute and are not curable. Therefore, continuity of care becomes an essential requirement, together with an appreciation of the whole person — not just his coronary arteries, or her uterus, or his blood pressure.

Specialists are wonderful, bless them. But for heaven's sake, first have a primary care doctor.

Is it time for a geriatrician?

I am often asked whether a geriatrician — a doctor who has a particular interest and competence in taking care of older patients — is an appropriate doctor to choose for an older person. In one sense, almost all doctors except pediatricians are geriatricians. Dermatologists, ophthalmologists, urologists, and orthopedists all have mostly gray-haired patients in their waiting rooms. Certainly most specialty internists also predominantly concern themselves with the healthcare needs of older persons.

Geriatrics is a special case. Unlike cardiology and the other medical "-ologies," no certifying specialty board exists for geriatrics. Instead, geriatricians receive a certificate for added competency, which both internists and family practitioners are eligible to seek through dedicated training programs and a probing examination. This certification serves as a sturdy reference indicating that the holder displays a special devotion to older persons. Less than 10,000 M.D.s hold this special diploma, however — not nearly enough to take care of even a fraction of the need.

I have never been a great fan of badges and degrees. Much more important are the inner qualities of the individual practitioner. Said in another way, I feel that labels are not as important as the end products. Physicians who do not call themselves geriatricians, but render the care without putting an identifying tag on it, deliver most older persons' medical care. Although Great Britain, particularly, has emphasized the role of geriatrics specialists in an older person's medical care, the fact remains that there are simply too many of us gray-headed folks around to be consigned to a small group of doctors. All M.D.s, except pediatricians, need to be geriatricians, diploma or not. Be sure to ask your doctor — or the nurse — about his background in working with older persons.

The qualities that really matter in a doctor for an older person are kindness, reliability, availability, knowledge, technical skill, and, yes, specialized training, if the doctor has acquired it. However, specialization is not on the what-matters-most list. Having a highly credentialed, brilliant, pleasant physician that is never available makes no sense.

The aptly named "physician extender"

Appreciation of the nurse's central helping role in the healthcare system has led to an extension of the nursing role. A new category of health professional, commonly called the "physician extender," has emerged and is growing rapidly. Physician extenders come in two varieties — nurse practitioners and physician's assistants. Each has different training and credentialing, but both play the same role: to augment the present system. Extra training for physician extenders allows increased competence. I've had extensive experience working with physician extenders and find them of huge value in making medical help more readily available to patients, particularly in geriatric medicine. You will be fortunate if the healthcare system or doctor's office you select contains physician extenders on its staff.

The role of the nurse

One of those really important secrets in the medical world is that the doctor's nurse is the most important member of your healthcare team. I'll take it one step further: Although the nurse probably gets his or her paycheck from the doctor and works under the doctor's direction, the nurse — not the doctor — really runs the show.

Every successful doctor has a nurse who keeps things shipshape. The nurse is such an important part of the medical practice that I suggest trying to get to know the nurse before the doctor. When you know the nurse's attitudes, work habits, congeniality, and skills, you will likely know the doctor's too. The best attributes to find in a nurse are

- ✔ The nurse is the one who makes order out of disorder.
- ✔ The nurse likely has more of a health focus than a disease focus.
- ✔ The nurse understands how details matter.
- ✔ The nurse gets things done on time.
- ✔ The nurse has an attitude of, "Of course I can; of course we will."
- ✔ The nurse is strongly positive and denies helplessness.
- ✔ The nurse cares.

Acknowledging that, in my opinion, the nurses I have worked with have done more good for my patients than I have doesn't hurt my vanity one bit. I'd like to think that my nurses, patients, and I work together well as a team, but after the dust settles, in my view, the nurse has been more important in the patient's well-being than I.

The role of the pharmacist

Your pharmacist makes up an important component in your healthcare team. A pharmacist is a highly skilled and educated health professional whose purpose is to see that your medication is appropriate. Side effects from drugs often arise, as noted in the package inserts and often on the pill bottle. Your pharmacist bears the primary responsibility for seeing that you are taking just the right medicine, in the right amount, at the right time, and for the shortest length of time possible. The doctor's office and the pharmacy ideally should be linked, but separate. Down the road, the doctor's office and the pharmacy will become more closely linked as the information systems technology improves. All sorts of common information will be more easily and safely accessible.

Communication with your pharmacist is key, especially because the number of drugs is growing and the opportunity for error increasing. Prescriptions don't always provide the answer to your medical problems, and, in fact, a doctor may give a prescription in error. A report from the prestigious Institute of Medicine of the National Academy of Science researched the errors in the medical systems and found them to be alarmingly high. Many are due to poor penmanship, others to careless copying, and still others to medication errors. In any case, the flood of new drugs is confusing and can create a situation in which what you and your physician presume that you are taking is not, in fact, what is in your best interest. To help keep errors to a minimum and to build a relationship with your pharmacist, review the following checklist:

- ✔ Have your pharmacist conduct a total review of your medications every six months.

- ✔ Ask about possible interactions with over-the-counter drugs or herbal preparations.

- ✔ Double-check when to take and when not to take your medications.

- ✔ Find out if there is a generic equivalent to the brand name drug you're taking.

Other health providers

Looking beyond the usual sources for medical care — hospitals, private physician offices, and clinics — can lead you to other wonderful sources for healthcare. I'll bet that the community in which you live contains many resources to serve you. Many of these are community agencies, such as the local health departments, the visiting nurse association, home healthcare agencies, nutritionists, physical and occupational therapists, and exercise instructors. The Alliance for Families and

Children (www.alliance1.org) does noble work all over the country as does the Red Cross (www.redcross.org), Salvation Army (www.salvationarmy.org), and others. The local senior center, the American Association of Retired People, YMCAs, religious institutions, and service agencies such as Rotary Club, Lions Club, and others can help you find the care you seek as well.

Just one or two phone calls can put you in contact with a wide range of helping services. Often a centralized information referral center exists that maintains lists of persons and services for your needs. Using these referral centers may or may not involve a fee to you. Ideally, your physician should be involved with this broader network to facilitate coordination of care.

What to Tell Your New Doctor

Congratulations! You've chosen a doctor. But to get the most out of your first visit, you should rehearse for it. Get your thoughts organized in advance so that you use your time most efficiently. Write down the most important issues and take notes during the visit. A patient's retention of what the doctor says during a visit is imperfect. For this reason, you may consider bringing a family member or friend — even a tape recorder is helpful.

As part of your health inventory, you should keep written records of these items:

- The dates of your different illnesses.
- Your laboratory reports.
- Your medications.
- Summary copies of your physical examination, complete with pertinent diagnoses.
- Your family medical history.
- Your immunization records.

The major aim in preparing thoroughly for a visit is to use your physician — and the time he or she spends with you — wisely. The average middle-aged person sees a doctor five times a year, and the older person more. These averages are only averages however. It is well-known that medical encounters tend to cluster. A relatively small number of persons, young and old alike, account for a disproportionate share of healthcare needs. In other words, most people are healthy.

Alternatives to the Doctor-Patient Model

There is an increasing emphasis to rely on self-management. *Self-management* means developing a greater awareness of the simple measures which you can safely institute without recourse to the doctor's office. These simple measures may include taking acetaminophen or aspirin, changing your diet, using a hot compress, or simply allowing time to heal. You have a responsibility to track your own health. The availability of more Internet services, including the ability to e-mail directly to your doctor's office, can help to reduce unneeded calls and visits. Estimates indicate that 30 to 50 percent of trips to the doctor's office are unnecessary. The better informed you become, the better patient you will be. Your health depends on you and your doctor together, but mostly on you.

Interest in group therapy is increasing. In group therapy, patients with similar conditions — such as asthma, arthritis, or chronic pain — work together with a health team. The support provided by group activities exceeds that of the usual one-on-one scenario.

Group sessions allow marvelous sharing of common experiences. Unexpected coping suggestions often emerge from others who are suffering from the same disease worries that you have.

Despite your best healthcare precautions, emergencies happen. You need to have a precise knowledge of what to do in an emergency. Your physician should guide you in determining what to do. When do you call 911 and when do you call the emergency room? How do you know when you should call? You don't want to call too quickly, but you certainly don't want to call too late. Knowing how to use your healthcare system is the key. Check out Chapter 11 to learn more about how to handle a healthcare crisis.

Taking a Health Exam

In recent years, many people have criticized the routine physical, claiming that it just isn't worth the expense. I disagree. If you argue that examining an otherwise healthy person is unduly expensive in comparison to the small amount of severe illnesses that such exams reveal, I agree. Few healthy people have serious and unsuspected diseases that a routine physical exam would uncover. However, everyone needs regular refresher courses on the best self-management strategies to stay well. This particularly holds true as people age, when small dietary, activity, or attitude readjustments here and there can induce major functional improvements. Blood pressure tests, mammographies, prostate checkups, osteoporosis assessments, nutritional and sleep pattern reviews, exercise estimates, cholesterol checks, prostate specific antigen test, blood sugar tests, and so forth may seem pretty mundane, but maintaining a general surveillance and record makes sure that the alarm bell of trouble does not ring suddenly.

Everyone over 60 years of age should have an annual health review, which includes a complete survey of current problems and habits including medication inventory, a physical exam, and appropriate lab tests. *Appropriate* is the key word here. Fortunately, doctors are evolving a sensible and defensible set of recommendations of how often people should perform certain tests. Over-testing is as bad as under-testing. The occasion of a physical exam also provides the opportunity to discuss other fundamental elements — among them sexuality, depression, balance, cognition, and memory changes. You should include a regular review of possible end-of-life scenarios. You need to apprise your physician of what you want done when you can no longer act independently on your own interests. A living will or a durable power of attorney for healthcare is a valuable document, but is not as important as you establishing with your doctor clear and unambiguous instructions about what you want to happen when.

Find a physician who sees the value of "routine" health exams, especially as you grow older. Sharing this sense of the value of preventive maintenance with your physician is key. Waiting until a warning symptom occurs is just plain too late, in my opinion.

Chapter 3

Exercising to Keep Your Health for Life

- -

In This Chapter

▶ Moving it or losing it: Exercise as the key component of health

▶ Learning what to exercise and how to exercise

▶ Opting not to exercise

- -

*H*ealth is something you may not fully appreciate until it's gone. We drink to each other's health; we teach children to be healthy, wealthy, and wise; and we all know that if you have health, you have everything. But what really is health? What are its components? How can we choose health over frailty, and what can we do today to ensure health for life? As Chapter 1 discusses, there are three main components to good health. This chapter delves into the first of those components: physical exercise. Chapters 4 and 5 discuss diet and relaxation to round out your physical-health plan!

Viewing Exercise as a Must, Not an Option

Exercise for the young is an option, but exercise for the old is a must. The reason for this, of course, is that young people possess a large margin of reserve from which they can withdraw their health benefits. Older people, however, possess a smaller health reserve. Older people need to build and maintain their health reserves — and exercise is a primary method to do so. People don't stop moving when they get old. People get old when they stop moving.

Exercise cuts down mortality rates at any age, but the protection grows increasingly stronger the older you become. One of the wonderful parts of life is its almost limitless capacity for resilience. Too often I hear, "if only I had started earlier," like jazz pianist Euby Blake's famous "I'd have taken better care of myself if I had known I would live this long." Fortunately for late entrants to the exercise world, the refrain is off-key. Even if people overdraw the health account by not exercising for several decades, they can still reverse their health with an exercise program. The message: Starting late is better than never starting at all!

How exercise can save your life

I have incorporated exercise into my life so that it is as integral as eating and breathing. If I ever miss a date in my exercise protocol, I feel like my pants are unzipped or I failed to brush my teeth. I am addicted to exercise.

I truly believe that exercise saved my life — and it can save yours, too. I had always actively participated in sports in high school and played intramural sports in college and squash and touch football in medical school. However, not until my dad died when I was 42 did I make exercise an end unto itself. My dad was a hero figure to me. I modeled what I did after him, even becoming a doctor like him. When he died, I cracked. I floundered. I couldn't work, think, or sleep. I was clinically depressed.

Why we're naturally averse to exercise

The roots of the human resistance to exercise run deep. All animals tightly balance the amount of movement that they undertake against the amount that they need to do to eat and reproduce. The truth is that all animals only move as much as they need to — period. (After all, the First Law of Thermodynamics does assert the conservation of energy.)

The anthropologists have a term for this resistance to exercise: "The Principle of Least Effort." Concisely stated, the principle observes, "Any creature, when having a task to perform, will select the way of performing the task that requires the least effort."

So, if you are a beaver building a dam, you select twigs and branches from your own valley, not one or two ridges away. If you are a hummingbird living in the Florida Keys with a girlfriend in Honduras, you select a straight flight route, not one that meanders around the Caribbean. Indeed, such a bird would tightly calculate the amount of fat he stores in his tanks to get him just the correct distance, with maybe a little bit extra in case he encounters head winds.

Today, humankind exploits the Principle of Least Effort to its highest degree. Need evidence? Look at the golf cart, electric carving knife, and electric toothbrush. At this rate, our poor muscles will have nothing left to do!

Then I started to run in a desperate effort to escape my grief. It worked. I have now been running for 28 years, a marathon a year. Three years ago, I added weight training and stretching to the program. As I write this, my wife and daughter just finished the Pike's Peak ascent, and I am planning on running the Boston Marathon shortly after my 70th birthday this year.

Why exercise is the ultimate prescription

Some people call exercise the universal therapy. They're right — exercise is good for just about everything. I recall, for example, when esteemed cardiologist Paul Dudly White encouraged President Dwight Eisenhower to get out on the golf course after his heart attack. Back in the 1950s, this advice constituted heresy. At the time, the standard medical treatment after a heart attack was 10 to 14 days in bed and another two weeks in the hospital. Terrible! Now, the American Heart Association even labels lack of exercise as one of the major causes of heart trouble. Exercise is a mandated part of the post-attack treatment phase. Exercise promotes healing and enables arteries to become bigger and better, helping to prevent another attack. The exercise prescription holds true not only for heart disease, but many other medical conditions. In fact, listing conditions in which you shouldn't exercise is much more difficult than nominating illnesses for which exercise is a healer.

The Fifty Plus Fitness Association

Fitness matters a lot, particularly as people age. A commitment to exercising led my wife and me to become avid supporters of the Fifty Plus Fitness Association. This group, 2,100 members strong across the country, was initiated at Stanford University 15 years ago in an effort to provide researchers with a group of fit older people to study the benefits of an active lifestyle. Today, 20 articles about our group have appeared in scientific literature. Researchers have scrutinized our bone density, fracture rate, sexuality, quality of life, and more. Dr. Jim Fries of Stanford recorded that our group of older exercisers, not elite by any standard, had mortality and disability rates that were 70 percent below the national average. I suggest that instead of the President or Congress convening any more blue ribbon panels to decide what to do about redesigning Medicare, they would be better served by simply mandating membership in the Fifty Plus Fitness Association. I hope that our number and our message grow. Check out the association's Web site at www.50plusfitness.org for more information.

Exercise is good for what ails you — including some cancers. Harvard alumni who exercised 2,000 calories per week (approximately 3 ½ hours of jogging or 7 hours of moderate-paced walking) had a 40 percent lower chance of developing prostate cancer. Since I found this out, my thrice-weekly jogs have a livelier bounce — now I know they are providing prostate health, too.

Every day, taboos against exercise are breaking down. Until recently, I felt that exercise was a no-no for patients with congestive heart failure — a condition in which a damaged heart simply doesn't pump adequately. Then a major scientific study from Italy appeared and showed the increased benefit of a walking program on a group of patients with congestive heart failure. Now, when we conduct research projects with older persons to seek out life quality benefits with exercise, we exclude virtually no one from participating in our walking programs. Walking is manifestly safe.

If a pill existed that provided all of the health benefits that exercise provides, the whole country would be on it.

Exercising with no competition pressure

Many people define what exercise is all about through sports and its competitive element. The competitive aspect intimidates some people and keeps them from exercising. But exercise and competition are not synonymous. True, many sports do involve exercise. However, many sports involve no exercise at all. Take a look at an issue of a popular sports magazine. You will find coverage of all sorts of events the magazine terms sports that involve no exercise whatsoever. Sports like croquet, archery, and bowling don't qualify as exercise. To my greatest dismay, golfing with a golf cart has descended virtually to the level of a spectator sport because the players barely exercise.

Don't get me wrong. Sports give an important boost to my quality of life. I read the sports section of the morning newspaper first, I wouldn't miss a Stanford football game, and I revere athletes for the thrills they provide. Exercise, however, is an on-board experience. You can't import energy flow from the newspapers or television, but taking a brisk walk, raking leaves, and riding your bike sure can give you an energy boost!

Use It Or Lose It: The Disuse Syndrome

In addition to all the braininess our species accumulated over the last 500 years (or 25 generations), it also developed a downside. I've made a list of six health conditions that are not due to bad genes, disease, or aging, but simply to disuse created by human laziness. I published this list as "The Disuse Syndrome" in the *Western Journal of Medicine* 10 years ago. In Chapter 1, I briefly mention this syndrome. These six, common ailments often occur as a group and originate from the same cause: sloth. A strange word, but, as one of the "seven deadly sins," a word that certainly describes our culturally induced laziness. The six health conditions that sloth and disuse cause are:

- ✔ Cardiovascular vulnerability
- ✔ Musculoskeletal fragility
- ✔ Immunologic susceptibility
- ✔ Obesity
- ✔ Depression
- ✔ Premature aging

The medical establishment hasn't given disuse syndrome the recognition that I think it deserves. However, the sooner people banish disuse by the simple strategy of increasing their exercise habits, the sooner they will regain the robust health that our ancestors handed down to us.

Cardiovascular vulnerability

What are the causes of our ongoing epidemic of heart disease — high cholesterol, high blood pressure, easy clottability, or lack of exercise? The answer is lack of exercise.

What are exercise's healthy heart credentials? It enlarges the arteries, it lowers total cholesterol while raising the good HDL cholesterol, and it lowers the blood pressure, thereby decreasing blood clots. Additionally, exercise reduces artery rigidity, improves heart contractility, increases capillary density, and lowers resting pulse rate.

Exercise should be your first resort, medicine your last resort. I attended a presentation by the chairman of the Stanford University Medical Center's division of cardiology at which he focused on the hopes and problems of gene therapy for heart disease. After looking at many slides and graphs, I raised my hand to ask: "Couldn't all of the above be achieved more efficiently, more cheaply, and more safely with exercise?" His answer: "Of course."

Musculoskeletal fragility

Muscles are made to move. Movement needs muscles to happen — or it used to anyhow. Our muscles and bones are frail caricatures of what they used to be. In the past, only the fittest survived. Now the fittest still survive, as do the weakest, but often in a dependent state. Dependency is the one element of growing older that holds most apprehension for people.

Dr. Mary Tinetti, professor of medicine, and her colleagues at Yale found the biggest predictor for an eventual need to go to a nursing home is lack of leg strength. This observation has led me to suggest that the most important part of the human body as it grows older is not the heart, lungs, kidneys, or liver, but the legs. As long as we keep our legs in working order, the rest of the machine tends to take care of itself. If the legs go, however, the ride is all downhill from there. Dependency lurks.

Immunologic susceptibility

Does the human ability to fight infection decrease as a natural part of aging, or does lowered physical activity create this problem? One of the stated definitions of aging is loss of resistance to infection. Is this the result of aging or of less physical activity? I have dozens of scientific papers in my files that demonstrate how the immune defenses go up in fit people and down in unfit people. Fit people just don't get sick as often as unfit people do. An active lifestyle stimulates a whole host of defense mechanisms that our bodies have developed to ward off infections, allergies, and maybe even cancer. I must mention, however, that overtraining (such as Olympic athletes at competition time) can put you at risk for infection. For every person who exercises too much, however, 10,000 people do not exercise enough — and suffer too many sick days as a result.

Obesity

Obesity in the United States has reached epidemic proportions. The Harvard School of Public Health conducted the most important experiment ever done in obesity research. Jean Mayer measured the food intake of a colony of rats that was living under ideal laboratory conditions. The rats, like animals in the wild, ate exactly the right amount of food. (Obesity does not exist in wild animals.) Then, Mayer raised the exercise of the animals by progressively increased amounts of 20 percent, 50 percent, and 150 percent. Without coaching, the rats increased their food intake by exactly the right amount so that they maintained a steady body weight.

The experiment didn't end there, though. Mayer then confined the free moving animals to small containers, limiting their exercise. The rats continued to eat the same amount as they were eating when they were active, and, consequently, became fat.

Our eating centers (located in the hypothalamus of our brains) were programmed 150,000 generations ago when our ancestors were busy as hunters and gatherers in Africa. Human obesity did not exist then. In fact, starvation was probably the rule of the day. Today, our eating centers remain as they have always been, but we, like the confined rats, have stopped moving, and we are getting fatter. Some surveys seem to indicate that for certain large groups of people, their intake is actually lower than it was for their ancestors in the past, yet the people are still fat. How come? Because of disuse. It is highly likely that the reason diabetes in the United States has increased from 1 million to 16 million cases in the past 40 years and continues to rise is because inactivity promotes obesity, which leads to diabetes. Genes haven't changed, but our activity pattern has.

Depression

Depression is common and often frequently unrecognized. Fortunately, depression often responds to a wide variety of antidepressant medicines we have in our doctors' bags. But is that medication the right or appropriate solution? Why does depression exist? When doctors analyze the brains of depressed people for their content of the catecholamines, such as norepinephrine and dopamine, they find them to be at low levels. These compounds are stimulators — the uppers of the neurotransmitters. So when the physician prescribes an antidepressant medicine, in effect he is providing a proxy, a substitute for solving the problem in a natural way, such as through exercise. Such substitution is similar to giving L-dopa to a patient with Parkinson's disease or insulin to a person with diabetes.

Does a natural way to increase the brain's catecholamine content exist? Of course. Exercise produces just the desired effect. The catechol levels rise shortly after the start of exercise. These catechols modulate a host of body changes that accompany exercise, such as the increased heart rate, sweating, higher blood sugar and fat transport, and production of endorphins. In fact, all of these body functions go up with exercise and down in depression, which has led many psychiatrists to incorporate an exercise prescription into their patients' treatment plans. Keith Jonsgaard wrote, "No depression is severe enough to withstand a 10-mile run." It follows naturally that if the whole world is underexercised, maybe the whole world is depressed. Maybe we should require all our leaders to take a 10-mile hike or jog before they deliberate our futures!

Premature aging

Disuse accelerates our aging process. Three-quarters of our aging would vanish if we remained fit. Exercising allows us to age and grow old naturally, rather than the feeble contemporary way we are now doing it. Exercise provides a 30-year age offset. A fit person of 70 corresponds biologically to an unfit person of 40. Exercise is the centerpiece of healthful aging.

You may have heard someone say, "Don't run up that hill or you'll use up some of your heartbeats." It's true that a trip up a hill does raise my pulse to 150 or so, but as I sit writing this, my pulse rate remains at a stately 45 beats per minute. Physical fitness is notable by its lowering of the resting pulse rate, and 45 beats per minute is evidence of a well-conditioned heart and body.

Exercising Your Way to a Healthier You

Okay, already! Exercise is good for you, from sex to serenity and from colon to cholesterol. So when do you start exercising? The answer, as always, is now. But first, you must understand the different types of exercise and how they can each benefit you. Exercise comes in four flavors, and you must include them all in your routine to receive the full benefit. (For a more complete look at different types of exercising, check out *Fitness For Dummies* and *Weight Training For Dummies,* both published by Hungry Minds, Inc.) The four types of exercise are:

- Aerobics
- Strengthening
- Flexibility
- Balance

Aerobic exercise

Of the four types of exercise, aerobics is the most crucial. Why? Because aerobics improves our ability to transport oxygen — our single most important bodily function. Like a candle under a glass tumbler, a person can live only four minutes without oxygen. A life extinguishes quickly when deprived of its oxygen. That's why how we handle oxygen is our most essential vital function.

The capacity to handle oxygen depends on the ability of our respiratory system to inhale oxygen from the atmosphere where it enters the lungs. From the lungs, the oxygen travels down to the hemoglobin of our red blood cells and through our circulatory system to every one of our 10 trillion cells. At the cells, the hemoglobin releases the oxygen to so that it can participate in that basic life chemical reaction — sugar plus oxygen yields carbon dioxide, water, and energy. Energy drives our metabolism, the machinery of life.

A fit person possesses well-oiled metabolic machinery that carries oxygen magnificently. An unfit person's oxygen carrying capacity is much less than in a fit person. Drs. Kasch and Boyer at San Diego State University have tracked the VO_2 values (oxygen transport capacity) of a group of fit and unfit men over 20 years. The fitness group's oxygen carrying capacity declined at a rate of 0.5 percent per year, whereas the unfit group lost its capacity at 2 percent per year. After 40 years, the yearly 1.5 percent difference gives the fit person a 60 percent better oxygen transport capacity than the unfit person. That's a huge difference! Additionally, Herb de Vries at USC showed that even 70-year-olds can improve their VO_2 max and become fit again.

What kinds of exercise yield aerobic benefit? Generally, aerobic exercises contain rhythmic and sustained motion — clear examples include walking at a rapid gate, jogging, swimming, biking, square dancing, aerobic dance, cross country skiing, and running. The aerobic value of other activities like racquet sports or soccer depends on the manner in which you play the sport. Some tennis or soccer players play so skillfully or indifferently that they raise no sweat. Others play in a clearly aerobic flowing, bouncy, rhythmic fashion. The two major sports of football and baseball clearly require an effort to become aerobic. (Many famous athletes are in lousy aerobic shape!)

Muscle strengthening

People are just now recognizing that being strong is a major health benefit. Some people disparage the muscle-builder physique. Once upon a time, I was one of those people until a friend confronted me about the long-term effects of not working all the important muscle groups — for example, not being able to lift my great-grandchildren when I am 85. Now I lift weights, and although my arms don't rival Arnold Schwarzenegger's, they'll certainly be ready to play with my great-grandchildren!

Certainly the biggest boon received by strength training is the knowledge that hip fractures and their predecessors of osteoporosis and sarcopenia (weak muscles) directly result from lack of muscle use. On the basis of mass alone, most of the body is muscle. Muscles serve a purpose, and if you don't use them, a gentle trip could lead you to a dangerous fractured hip.

A little digging reveals even sturdier credentials in support of strength training than merely the prevention of hip fractures. Being strong helps circulation, metabolism, nerve conduction, bowel and bladder control, self image, weight management, and joint stability. Strength is a major asset to the person with arthritis, because well-tended ligaments and muscles hold the joint in place, lowering the likelihood of injury and disability.

Improving your strength may seem intimidating, but it isn't. Strength training requires only minimal equipment, doesn't cost much, and can be done anywhere. Many people find that health clubs and gyms help in the strengthening effort by supplying social support and a variety of equipment. Still, you don't need a gym to do strength training — you can work out right in your own home, which we'll talk about later in this chapter.

Becoming strong is very safe if you use your head. The saying, "No pain, no gain" is a hazard. "No brain, no gain" is more like it. If you experience pain, you should stop what you're doing. The smarter you are about developing your strengthening program, the better it will work for you.

You should work at strengthening the whole body. Your program should involve the chest, abdomen, and back, as well as the arms (shoulders, biceps, triceps, and wrists), and legs (quads, hamstrings, and ankles). I define the particulars of this effort later in this chapter, but for now, know that the rest of your life will be healthier if you build and maintain a good set of muscles. You can't start too late!

Flexibility

Loss of elasticity is one of the marks of aging. The pinch test of the skin on the back of the hand proves this. The pinch test consists of pinching the back of a person's hand: on a younger person, the skin snaps back to its usual place; on an older person, the skin remains in a tent position for several seconds. Certainly aging does create stiffness and impermeabilities due to free radical damage to the collagen tissue, but disuse compounds such damage. Witness how miserable a casted leg becomes. In a cast, a leg becomes stiff and withered, not because it ages, but because you can't stretch it.

As part of my fitness program, I do a set of stretches to my neck, shoulders, back, belly, and hips during my thrice-weekly strengthening program. The stretches are nothing too extreme, just enough to help me maintain an exclamation point posture (think straight up-and-down) and avoid the comma posture (think hunched) that I see too often in older persons. You need to work at it to remain flexible. Stretching also boasts particularly strong credentials as a stress buster. Almost nothing releases stress as well as a generous stretch. When you're stressed, you tense up — just as an animal does under threat. Your muscles tighten like a bowstring. The tightening, particularly if protracted, wears you out too soon.

Most of the advisories about strengthening also apply to stretching. Stretching certainly requires no equipment and should be totally safe if you don't overdo it by bouncing or pushing yourself into a painful state. Bouncing to stretch leads to overstretching and injury.

Stretching should involve two stages: first, an easy and totally natural stage, and second, a slight extension. The stretch should gradually release tension as you hold the position. Again, all parts of the body should have their own protocol.

I highly recommend yoga, tai chi, and ch'i gung for both flexibility and balance training. Check out your local fitness club or YMCA to see if you can sign up for classes in these areas. Any person experienced in these exercises gains a major health advantage in muscle and joint flexibility.

Balance

Balance training sits at the end of the list of exercise goals. This category only recently joined the other components of exercise training, because, until people started growing older in large numbers, doctors didn't recognize balance as an issue.

Balance, like swallowing, is a complex neuromuscular event that we take for granted. We don't consciously think about swallowing or balance, but when one or the other becomes defective, we recognize what a critical role it plays. Balance depends on a whole hierarchy of events starting at the head and reaching to the toes. The brain, the eyes, the inner ear, the spinal column, the muscles, and the many position sense receptors all constantly work together to inform us of our body location and position. The efficiency of this gyroscope function is superb, but when it gets tipsy, the effect seriously impairs your quality of life.

Too often the first recognition of bad balance comes after a fall. Clearly, this realization arrives too late. So I advocate that all of us involved in the process of growing older incorporate the fourth training module into our exercise schedule. Usually, this module works easily with a strengthening and stretching routine so that you cover all of the exercise bases. Like the other exercises, balance training requires no equipment, fancy clothing, or gear.

Together, aerobics, strengthening, flexibility, and balance constitute the blueprint for vigor. The next section explores the "hows" of exercise — how much, how hard, and how often.

Deciding on an Exercise Program that's Right for You

Now that you know the elements of exercise, you need to make a plan. The first question to answer is, how much should you exercise? The Greeks advised, "Everything in moderation," which still holds true today. However, the truth about exercise is that for every one person who does too much, thousands of others do too little. Those of us in the health professions worry less about people exercising in moderation than about people not exercising at all!

A great real-life example of the proportion of people who choose to exercise enough is to watch people approach the escalator in an airport. For every one person who walks or climbs, 30 to 40 people stand and ride — the Principle of Least Effort rears its ugly head again. I have validated this ratio over and over. At lectures I give around the country, I often describe these findings, and then delight to find more people on the stairs than on the elevator and escalator after the lecture ends.

Steve Blair, at the Aerobic Center in Dallas, found that the most important increment of exercise is the first. That is, a little exercise for the sedentary person provides more benefits than a little more exercise for the already-active person. Recently, the Surgeon General's Report on Exercise, of which Steve was the lead author, emphasized light exercise, such as raking leaves, as the primary national goal. While light exercise is a good start — and the report probably gave it as a suggestion so as not to intimidate first-time exercisers — the truth is the more exercise, the better. Walking, running, or stair climbing provide many more benefits. As always, if you've recently been under a doctor's care for a heart attack, high fever, or persistent pain, you should check with your doctor first before beginning any exercise program.

You can measure how much you should exercise in several ways. One is calorie count. Calories are units of energy. Table 3-1 shows you the number of calories you expend in several common activities.

Table 3-1	Calories per hour for 150 lb. person	
	Men	*Women*
Walking	300	250
Jogging	500	350
Hard housework	400	250
Tennis	500	400
Golfing (cart)	250	200
Running	700	500

You can also use a unit of measurement called a "met" to measure exercise. A "met" describes the intensity of different exercises, starting with one. One represents the amount of exercise you expend at rest. Some exercises can reach 10 mets, as you can see in Table 3-2. Every met is a multiple of a resting expenditure.

Table 3-2	Mets
Sitting	1
Walking	4
Running	6
Hard housework	8
Heavy weight lifting	10

Both calorie and met measurements represent exercise amounts that you must multiply by the time you spend doing them. A short, intense exercise may equal the calorie or total mets of a lesser intense exercise over a longer period.

Walking (at 270 calories an hour for a 150-pound person, or four mets) takes billing as the most common exercise. Walking is a low intensity exercise that adds up. While a pedometer — an instrument that records steps — attached to an inactive person might register 2,000 steps per day, an active schoolteacher's pedometer could register 7,000. The effectiveness of walking depends on how hard and how long you do it.

Another technique people use to measure the intensity of an exercise is pulse rate. Every one of us has a target pulse rate for which we should aim to achieve the maximum benefit from exercising. Our heart can beat only so fast no matter how hard we exercise. Doctors describe the maximum pulse rate as 220 minus your age. For me, at age 70, my calculations show that the fastest my heart can go, no matter how hard I push, is 150 beats per minute. The target pulse rate for aerobic exercise equals 70 percent of the maximum calculation — roughly 105 for my age mates and me.

Using the calorie count method relates the exercise amount to your diet, which certainly has value for some people. Simpler, but less revealing, is the pulse-rate technique, which tries to get to the same point, but uses the pulse as the indicator of intensity. Whichever technique you use to judge the intensity and length of your exercise plan is less important than doing it — and the worksheets at the end of this chapter will help you get started!

Setting targets and creating a program

How much exercise you should do depends first on how hard and how long. How hard can be measured in calories, mets, or pulse rate. Using these three intensity measurements, you should aim for levels that equal 10 calories, or 5 mets, or 130 pulse rate and sustain this intensity for 30 minutes. You should do this three times per week, minimum. Exercising four days per week benefits you even more than three, and five is better still, but exercising aerobically more than four times a week may be overdoing it and can increase your chance for injury.

Exercising for half an hour is a good start. A half-hour of activity realizes most, if not all, of the benefits of exercise, yet still fits into your daily schedule. Exercising for more than a half-hour probably brings more benefits, but you should clearly observe your upper limit. Remember, however, that for every one person who exceeds the upper limit, many, many more people never even approach this limit. Again, the greatest danger for most of us lies in underexercising, not overexercising!

You should strive to make your strengthening, stretching, and balance program not too much or too little, but just enough. If you'd prefer to do your strength training at home rather than join a gym, you need three things: ankle weights, bars with weights, and a sturdy comfortable bench — period. Before you start, some basic guidelines include:

- ✔ Go slow.
- ✔ Be consistent.
- ✔ Maintain good posture.
- ✔ Keep breathing.
- ✔ Use both sides of your body.
- ✔ Don't hurt yourself.

For strengthening, you should use enough weight for each individual muscle group (take a look at the sample worksheet at the end of this chapter for examples of exercises), so that at the end of eight repetitions of the movement, you feel moderate fatigue. As your strength increases, you need to increase the weight that you use for your arms, chest, and legs. Start with eight repetitions, done slowly. Group them into three sets of eight with a half or whole minute rest in between. To work each muscle group, you'll need to do 10 different exercises (three for the torso, three for the legs, and four for arms).

Your stretching routine should include the neck, back, sides, shoulders, and legs. Use the two-stage stretch — stretch the joint to its easy limit and then go about 5 percent to 10 percent beyond that — holding each stretch for 15 seconds, then repeating several times. Stretching is best done after some warm up, such as jogging in place, and again, should not be abrupt, jerky, or bouncy.

For the balancing portion of your routine, I suggest the flamingo stand, which consists simply of standing on one leg without any other support for 20 seconds. Then, change legs. It sounds easy, but give it a try — it will surprise you by how difficult it can be! If you can't do this exercise, you may hang on to the back of a chair with one hand or one finger to steady yourself until your balance improves. This exercise may not be the most exciting, but by mastering it, you could avoid a hip fracture.

When you get good at the flamingo stand, try it with your eyes closed.

Don't forget that any increase in your exercise effort, of whatever kind, will likely cause new soreness as you place your system under a new burden. You should expect such soreness, and, if you are an exercise addict as I am, you may think it almost feels good — like a badge of new accomplishment. If soreness lingers, or progresses, however, you need to reevaluate. But for most novice exercisers, soreness is not a reason to stop.

Scheduling your exercise routine

I find that exercising aerobically three times per week, a half hour each time, works with alternate days for strengthening, stretching, and balancing exercises. That way, you exercise six days a week, with one day of rest.

Your composite exercise program might look like:

- ✔ Something aerobic — Monday, Wednesday, Friday
- ✔ SSB (strength, stretch, balance) — Tuesday, Thursday, Saturday
- ✔ Sunday — off

At what time of the day you exercise is not critical, although first thing in the morning offers many advantages (this works best for me), such as:

- ✔ It gets rid of the cobwebs.
- ✔ The rest of the day hasn't had a chance to start crowding in.
- ✔ The telephone is less likely to ring.
- ✔ The rest of the day carries a natural high with it.
- ✔ Meal times are less likely to become cramped by exercise routines.

Use any or all of the preceding list to establish your best time of day routine.

Excuses, including inclement weather, travel, other opportunities, most illnesses, jet lag, and so forth, do not count! You must make exercise top priority. Exercise is the universal antidote to what ails us. And don't forget, the time is never too soon or too late to start. After all, life is the one race you win by finishing last.

At the end of this chapter, you'll find a sample "Getting Started" worksheet that will help you begin your exercise program. Notice the variety of exercises and also the consistency of activity — there's an activity almost every day! You'll also find a blank worksheet for you to use to develop your own workout plan. Please feel free to photocopy this worksheet so that you can reuse it and share it with your friends!

Getting Started: The Exercise Program That's Right for You!

Sample Weekly Workout Log for Week Beginning _____

	Monday	Tuesday	Wednesday	Thursday	Friday	Saturday	Sunday
Cardio Exercises							
Activity: Duration:	Power Walking 50 minutes				Power Walking 50 minutes		
Activity: Duration:		Bicycling 50 minutes		Bicycling 50 minutes			
Muscle Strength Exercises							
Activity: Duration:	Free Weights/ Upper Body 3 sets of 10 reps 5 different exercises		Free Weights/ Upper Body 3 sets of 10 reps 5 different exercises				
Activity: Duration:		Bent Knee Push-Ups 2 sets of 25		Bent Knee Push-Ups 2 sets of 25			
Activity: Duration:			Ab Crunches 2 sets of 25		Ab Crunches 2 sets of 25		
Flexibility Strength Exercises							
Activity: Duration:	Yoga 45 minutes			Yoga 45 minutes			
Activity: Duration:		Total Body Stretching Exercises 30 minutes					

Getting Started: The Exercise Program That's Right for You!

Weekly Workout Log for Week Beginning _____

	Monday	Tuesday	Wednesday	Thursday	Friday	Saturday	Sunday
Cardio Exercises							
Activity: Duration:							
Activity: Duration:							
Muscle Strength Exercises							
Activity: Duration:							
Activity: Duration:							
Activity: Duration:							
Flexibility Strength Exercises							
Activity: Duration:							
Activity: Duration:							

Chapter 4

Fueling Your Future with Good Food!

*P*roper diet, along with exercise and rest, is one of the three components of health. I often am asked, "As we age, what is the right diet?" My answer is always, a well-balanced, diverse diet is best — whatever age you are. You've probably seen the food pyramid, which is accepted as gospel by most nutrition experts. That's the perfect example of diversity in your diet, and if you follow the pyramid, then you're home safe. You don't need any fancy cookbooks or kooky diets. You just have to eat smart. Being smart about the food you put in your mouth is a major part of living long.

In this chapter, I provide a summary of the basic info for you, the present and future agers, to stash away and use the next time you are at the store, or in the kitchen, or at the dinner table. I supply the fundamentals, the whats, the how tos, the whys, and the whens that should lead to healthy choices. We are fortunate to be alive when so many food choices are available, but unless you make these choices wisely, food can become your enemy instead of your friend.

You Are What You Eat

The saying, "You are what you eat" is inescapably true. Your food makes up your anatomy. Although the image your mirror reflects today looks pretty similar to the one you saw last year, the truth is that you are almost entirely new — newly constituted from the raw material of the thousand meals that you ate over the last year.

Food is more than just your structure. Food is your energy source. Not only does your food provide your structure, it also supplies the fuel to run that structure, to do what you want and need to do. When you look at nutrition over your life span, you need to consider both the structure-building and energy-generating properties of food.

Eating your way through 75 million calories

Over a 100-year lifetime, you eat around 75 million calories. That's enough food to feed the entire hungry crowd at the Super Bowl. Calories are divided into three parts: carbohydrate, protein, and fat. Each is different chemically. Carbohydrate and fat are each comprised of three elements: carbon, hydrogen, and oxygen. Protein, on the other hand, contains these three plus nitrogen, sulfur, and phosphorus. Carbohydrate and fat serve almost exclusively as energy sources. Protein serves almost exclusively as structure, the "meat" of us.

Dietary carbohydrate is the short-term energy supplier, fat is the long-term energy source, and protein is structure. The body's machinery breaks them down to the same small two-carbon molecule before they are combusted for energy. The same little molecule also serves as the building block for fat formation. This explains why a person may become fat when eating too much carbohydrate, too much fat, or too much protein. All three can make you fat, but eating fat will make you fat faster because it is so rich in calories compared with the other two.

Dietary building blocks

The U.S. Department of Agriculture food pyramid, shown in Figure 4-1, emphasizes variety in the diet. The emphasis is on vegetables, fruits, and grains. For more information on these important components to your diet, refer to *Nutrition For Dummies* (Hungry Minds, Inc.).

You'll notice that the food pyramid doesn't acknowledge the great American sweet tooth. People in the United States consume 156 pounds of sugar per person per year, and this figure has risen substantially in recent years. Not only does this high sugar consumption result in more calories, but also those calories are "empty" — this means that foods such as sweets, particularly candy and sodas, have no value other than calories.

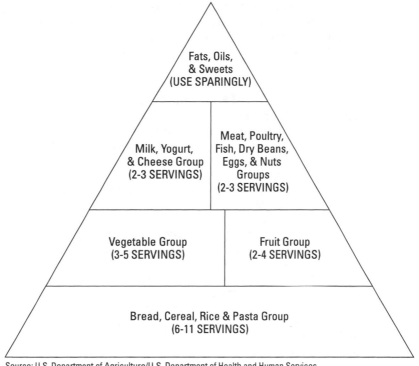

Fats, Oils,
& Sweets
(USE SPARINGLY)

Milk, Yogurt,
& Cheese Group
(2-3 SERVINGS)

Meat, Poultry,
Fish, Dry Beans,
Eggs, & Nuts
Groups
(2-3 SERVINGS)

Vegetable Group
(3-5 SERVINGS)

Fruit Group
(2-4 SERVINGS)

Bread, Cereal, Rice & Pasta Group
(6-11 SERVINGS)

Source: U.S. Department of Agriculture/U.S. Department of Health and Human Services

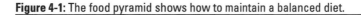

Figure 4-1: The food pyramid shows how to maintain a balanced diet.

Protein

Protein is an important part of our balanced diet and should constitute 15 to 20 percent of our daily calories. I think protein should definitely form a major part of our diet as we age. In the past, protein has gotten a bad rap. One argument against protein was that with kidney disease, the breakdown products of protein pile up in the blood, which leads to uremia, meaning too many toxic nitrogen compounds in the blood. But when the kidneys are healthy, they are very capable of getting rid of all waste that is generated.

The main problem with protein, however, is that we get most of it from meat, and meat contains fat. There's no question that marbling — the distribution of fat in meat — increases the flavor and accounts for much of the appeal of steaks, roasts, chops, and burgers. There are several important reasons to limit the overall intake of fat, particularly animal fat. This consideration makes awareness of other good sources of dietary protein, such as soy foods, egg whites, and reduced fat milk, even more important. Still, meat serves as a prime source for protein, and we need to be sure that our intake of protein is adequate to keep rebuilding ourselves over an entire life span. We keep growing and replacing until we die, and so we need protein until we die.

Fat

How much fat we need corresponds to how much fuel we need. As we age, our need for fuel depends on how active we remain. In my view, there is no difference in advice about fat to a 40-year-old or a 90-year-old. If you are physically active at 90 and your cholesterol level is satisfactory, you don't need to worry about the amount of fat you eat. If you are inactive, and/or your cholesterol is high, you should restrict your fat intake (I speak more on cholesterol later in this chapter). And, the same advice holds true for a 40-year-old.

For most of us, common sense about fat intake should prevail. I buy into the American Heart Association guidelines of 30 percent max of daily calories should be derived from fat — and preferably, that fat should come from the plant or unsaturated fats, such as olive oil, peanuts, and fish. To calculate the percentage of fat calories you are eating, you need to do a little figuring. First, you need to know the total number of calories you are eating. Either you can do this yourself by picking up a nutrition book at the library and scanning it, or by submitting your diet diary to a nutritionist who can calculate for you. Second, from the food list you consume, select those items which are the fatty containers, such as meats and cheeses. An ounce of meat, fried fish, or cheese contains, on average, 70 calories of fat. A cup of whole milk has 45 calories of fat, as does a teaspoon of oil or margarine, butter, or one slice of bacon. Adding up the day's intake of fat calories, divided by the total calories, yields the percentage. For instance, say your total calories come to 2000, and included in these are two pieces of bacon and a teaspoon of butter at breakfast, a slice of luncheon meat and cheese at lunch, and one six-ounce hamburger for dinner. These foods would yield 645 fat calories or roughly 32 percent of your day's calories are derived from fat.

You can eat marbled red meats and dairy products in moderation, but these contain saturated fats, and you must be careful. Believe me, I understand the temptation. Cheese and ice cream are my own personal problems! I use my running program as an excuse to indulge myself occasionally.

Carbohydrate

Carbohydrate should be the main component of the day's fuel. Carbs should make up 50 percent max of your daily calories. Similar to the fat calculations mentioned earlier, to figure out the percentage of carbs that make up your total calorie intake, first, sort out the carbo foods, such as grains, veggies, and fruits. One cup's worth of cereal, pasta, or veggies, two slices of bread, a four-inch apple, or whole grapefruit all contain approximately 120 calories. Adding up the daily carbo foodstuffs and then dividing by your total calorie intake provides the percentage of carbohydrates that make up your daily calories.

Carbohydrate comes in three sizes: small, medium, and large. Small carbohydrates are the simple sugars, such as table sugars. Medium carbohydrates are two of the little ones linked up — fruit sugars are of this sort. Big carbohydrates are many little sugars linked together in a lattice work — the starches of grains and vegetables are of this sort.

The difference between carbohydrates derives from the ease with which they are absorbed. To enter the blood stream from the intestine, all types of carbohydrates must be converted to the small type. So, after they enter the blood, carbohydrates are all small. A potato or an orange after it is absorbed looks just the same as a lump of sugar after it's absorbed.

However, the rate of absorption varies according to the size of the carbohydrate and affects how quickly the body reacts to it. A big slug of a rapidly absorbed, small carbohydrate means that a big slug of insulin will be released. On the other hand, a big carbohydrate as it is slowly absorbed, takes longer to be released as insulin. Insulin, which is the important hormone made by your pancreas, is secreted in response to a rise in blood sugar after eating carbohydrates.

For this reason, big, complex carbohydrates are recommended by nutritionists. The other reason that grains and vegetables are favored fuels is that they carry with them other nutrients such as vitamins, minerals, and fiber. Table sugar, on the other hand, is an "empty" calorie because nothing else — no vitamins, minerals, or fiber — comes in with it. It is energy, true, but that's all, and its small size creates a blood sugar surge with a consequent insulin reaction. That reaction leads sometimes to reactive hypoglycemia, a period of weakness and shakiness two or three hours after a high carbohydrate sugar meal.

One of the main carbohydrate-related aging issues concerns milk. One of milk's chief nutrients is lactose, a medium-sized carbohydrate. For lactose to be absorbed, you must have an enzyme in the intestinal wall called lactase, which breaks the medium carbohydrate into two smaller carbohydrates. In many older people, the level of lactase goes down and the lactose cannot be absorbed. Instead, the lactose acts as a laxative, resulting in diarrhea and cramping. Some ethnic groups, particularly Asians, lack this enzyme from birth, and are limited in their dairy intake. Other ethnic groups tend to tolerate milk early in life, but may have trouble later on.

If you suspect you may have an intolerance to milk products, you can either avoid them, take them in smaller amounts, or you may elect to seek out over-the-counter lactase compounds.

The Catalysts

A catalyst is a facilitator, a helper, a promoter, which allows a chemical reaction. A vitamin acts as a catalyst and is critical in allowing the fuel (carb, fat, protein) to burn, but itself is not consumed in the process, but is instead regenerated to be used over and over again.

Vitamins

Micronutrients — vitamins and minerals — are as essential as macronutrients — protein, fat, and carbohydrate. Without micronutrients, a whole assortment of deficiency conditions may arise, from anemia to nerve problems.

Older people are at particular risk of vitamin or mineral underconsumption for a variety of reasons. There may be dental problems that affect chewing capacity, or some other economic, psychological, or social issues. Too often older persons' diets become unvarying. One of the basic tenets of good nutrition is variety, and that holds true for older people, too.

I advocate a multivitamin with minerals each day for my older patients. They are safe, cheap, and can help avoid lots of problems. Keep in mind, however, that vitamins are not a substitute for a good, balanced food program.

Minerals

Salt, calcium, and iron are the most important minerals. Our needs for minerals don't change as we age. Throughout life, salt should be used moderately. Luckily, the kidney, that wonder organ, usually compensates for under- or over-salting of food. If we eat too little salt, the kidney dams up salt in its excretion, and if we take in too much, it simply gets rid of it. Some people, particularly overweight people, are sodium retainers, which puts a person at risk for the development of high blood pressure.

Calcium is the stuff of our bones. Most of us have heard about the epidemic of osteoporosis — the reduction of bone density. The recommended intake is 1.5 grams of calcium per day — that's the amount of calcium you'll find in two glasses of milk!

Although low intake of calcium over a lifetime is a major cause of osteoporosis, insufficient exercise is a much bigger part of the problem (see Chapter 3 for details on exercise).

Iron is mostly important as part of our hemoglobin in the red blood cells. Generally a well-balanced diet provides enough iron for all purposes. Meats and green vegetables are excellent sources of iron.

Fiber

Fiber is often lacking in older people's diets, and it is difficult to compensate for by taking a pill. Plenty of fiber helps you to avoid constipation and to control cholesterol levels. Fiber, of course, is found largely in grains and vegetables, but if you can't seem to get enough fiber in your diet, you can take it in a prepared, drug store form.

Fluid

A word about fluid and aging. A few reports suggest that older people lose their thirst sensitivity, so remembering to drink liquids is important, particularly in hot weather. Sometimes if you rely on thirst to be your indication that you need a glass of water, it is already too late, and you are dehydrated. Be sure that your daily fluid intake adds up to two quarts.

Starting Out: The Best Food Plan for You

Now that you know the basics about food and nutrition, the time has come to talk a little more specifically about developing good eating habits. Any consideration of what is the right diet for you begins with the simple determination of how many calories you need to provide enough fuel for your furnace. I can't give you a snap answer to this query, because a person's size and their activity pattern determine each individual's calorie needs. Some people can maintain their body weight and strength on 1,500 calories per day. Others may not gain weight even on 5,000 calories per day.

The best diet plan is one that provides you with a little bit of everything you need for life. No fancy strategies or new discoveries offer a magic solution. This section fills you in on the building blocks of a good diet plan and helps you to discover what you need to eat to be fit for life.

What you should eat

Despite repeated pronouncements from the diet hucksters about such and such diet being the "best," "quickest," "brainiest," "sexiest," or "strongest," all these recipes are pure baloney. The definition of a good diet is maybe too simple. It is "enough, but not too much, of the basic nutrients." This means sufficient but not excessive calories, regardless of source, and then a sufficient mixture of foods from the basic food groups specified in the familiar pyramid to assure an adequate complement of the daily requirements of amino acids, unsaturated fatty acids, fiber, fluids, and micronutrients of vitamins and minerals. A terrific place to start in rethinking your food plan as you age is *Nutrition For Dummies* (Hungry Minds, Inc.), which expands greatly on these general guidelines and provides a number of fun recipes for your consideration.

How and when you should eat

How and when you consume food is almost as important as what you consume. Some people are said to be gorgers — a little or no breakfast, a sandwich and soft drink for lunch, and a monster meal in the evening. Other people are nibblers, meaning that they eat little bits all day long.

Being a nibbler is valuable for two reasons. First, cholesterol levels are lower in people who nibble rather than gorge. Second, it leads to a more stable and helpful blood sugar level. The blood sugar fluctuates throughout the day in response to the previously eaten food. To eat only once per day leads to a single big jump in the sugar instead of the more constant level of the nibbler.

Dieters, it doesn't matter how often you eat — it has no affect on weight loss. Thirty years ago, our research group in Philadelphia did an experiment in our nutrition study unit in which we fed dieters the same low-calorie formula, provided either as a single meal, three meals, or in eight, small, equal feedings. The rate of weight loss was the same regardless of the schedule, so we calculated that calories, and not their timing, was what determines the rate of weight loss. But, eating smaller amounts throughout the day is still considered a valuable eating habit.

Certainly, a huge part of eating well depends on how well you plan. At the end of this chapter, you'll find a "Getting Started" worksheet sample as a reference and a blank worksheet for you to develop your own plan. As with all the other worksheets in this book, feel free to photocopy it so that you can reuse it and share it with your friends!

Losing Weight

Even if you're very careful about what you eat and you try to exercise regularly, you may still feel like you need to drop a few pounds to feel healthy. Keep in mind, however, that losing weight is big business. Just go to the bookstores or health food stores and survey the mass of materials provided for the millions of people who seek relief from their tight pants. Unfortunately, almost all of these provide a gimmick. *Dieting For Dummies* (Hungry Minds, Inc.) cuts out all of this hoopla, and tells it like it is, no shortcuts, no miracle cures, just discipline and hard work, plus intelligence. Smart people live longer, and one of the reasons they do is that they eat better. The following guidelines should help you get jump-started.

Calories do count

Losing weight is not only good for your self-esteem, but it may also save your life. During research at the metabolic unit at the Lankenau Hospital in Philadelphia, other researchers and myself studied dozens of people, but far and away the most memorable of these was a young man who weighed 691 pounds. He stayed in our research unit for two years and participated in numerous projects. When he left he weighed 179 pounds — that's a weight loss of 512 pounds! I recorded his case in an article in the *American Journal of Medicine* entitled "A Five Hundred Pound Weight Loss." Recently I was able to track him down via the Internet and was delighted to find that he was still alive, married, and father to two children. He now weighs around 300 pounds (after having been up and down in weight several times), and he has heart trouble. But he is still alive, which he certainly would not have been had we not had the opportunity to study and help him. Combining our experience with dozens of obese research subjects, we concluded that calories do indeed count, and that the rate of weight loss observed under tightly controlled conditions was precisely predictable, a conclusion which I used in another paper I wrote, "The Predictability of Weight Loss" in the *Journal of the American Medical Association.* A pound of fat, my fat, your fat, bacon fat, contains 3500 calories. So whenever a pound is gained or lost, it means that this number has been either added or subtracted.

Exercise and activity patterns

If you haven't already heard enough about the benefits of exercise, here's another reason to start: as long as you remain physically active, you have great tolerance in the amount of calories you can consume. An active person can eat just about anything in any amount he or she desires, but when that person is inactive, all bets are off.

You have three choices:

- ✔ Exercise enough and eat what you want.
- ✔ Don't exercise and diet.
- ✔ Don't exercise, don't diet, and get fat.

Why the United States is fighting an obesity epidemic

The fact that people in the United States are becoming fatter is abundantly clear. The National Heart, Lung, and Blood Institute estimated in 1998 that 97 million people in the U.S. (55 percent of the population) are obese. That number has gone up 8 percent in 10 years. And I hate to imagine what the numbers will be like 10 years from now. These statistics are particularly troubling when viewed in connection with the growing number of older people in the U.S. (for more on this topic, see Chapter 1). The older body has less lean body tissue and more body fat, worsening the obesity problem.

Is the primary culprit for this obesity more food, less exercise, or a combination of the two? I believe the culprit is less exercise. Food consumption in the U.S. is actually recorded to be less than it was 10 years ago. Inactivity has thrown our bodies' eating control mechanisms out of whack, and as a result, people aren't burning off enough calories.

Are you overweight or obese? One of the simplest measures is just taking a look at your waist size. For a male of average height, 40 inches and up is too much. For a female of average height, 35 is maximum. A still simpler test is to look in the mirror. If you are honest, this examination is the only one you really need to heed the signal.

Exercise is the most important dietary advice. The answer to the question, "How much should I eat?" leads to another question, "How much do you exercise?" You need a certain amount of food just to keep your body's "pilot light" going, and beyond that you need calories to move. Chapter 3 gives caloric values for different types of exercise, so you can estimate your total. A big sports utility vehicle eats more gas than a subcompact car. The same principle goes for people.

When you embark on an exercise program, your body reacts by releasing a growth hormone to stimulate muscle growth. This means the scale might show that you are gaining weight or losing very little weight. However, this weight change is just an illusion, and because the muscle gain phase of diet and exercise is brief, you should see the scale start moving downward again in just a few days.

Shifting fluid

The main confounder of weight change is fluid shift. Fluid, or water, weighs a lot. Because one quart of water weighs 2.2 pounds, relatively minor shifts in water balance can cause big swings on the scale. Take comfort in the fact that such fluid shifts are temporary and will even out in the long run. When you're trying to lose weight, however, great consternation may result when the needle on the scale goes the opposite way from which you, the dieter, desire. Because of these water weight fluctuations, weighing yourself only once a week is a good idea — any more frequently will make you crazy!

Potentially Bad Stuff: Coffee, Soft Drinks, Alcohol, and Cholesterol

While I've spent a lot of this chapter talking about all the important, good things that you should be eating and drinking as fuel for your body, some of the bad things are worth a mention so that you can try to steer clear from them whenever possible. Lots of different drinks have plenty of caffeine in them, which can make you jittery and disrupt your sleep patterns. Alcohol has plenty of bad side effects when consumed in large amounts, and there are good and bad kinds of cholesterol to consider. Read on!

Coffee and soft drinks

People love coffee. Coffee is how many people start their days, and it provides the perfect excuse for a break during the day. The only substantial rap I have against coffee is caffeine's ability to jazz us up, which of course is the very reason that people drink coffee. Often, however, our lives are so jazzed up already that coffee may make the world spin too fast. Fortunately, our bodies develop a tolerance to caffeine, so the over-stimulation effect is blunted after a short while. Another potential negative to coffee is the tendency of caffeine to dehydrate us.

The United States is on a soft drink binge, which seems to be growing worse and worse. The U.S. consumption of pop is measured in super tanker amounts annually. The central problem is, of course, that the great majority of sodas provide almost no nutritive value. They do give us sugar, but do we need more sugar in our lives? Some nutritionists even blame soft drinks for the obesity epidemic. Diet soft drinks omit the sugar but contain salt and often contain caffeine, which lack nutritive value. Water is cheaper and safer.

Alcohol

Alcohol is a problem for many people — and as we age, the problem doesn't go away. A recent survey of the drinking habits of 4,000 people over 65 revealed that 79 percent of them were consuming some alcohol. Twenty-five percent (31 percent of men, and 19 percent of women) drank daily. Fifteen percent of those who drank were considered to be heavy drinkers, equally distributed between the two sexes. Binge drinking was not uncommon, as 10 percent of the drinkers reported five or more drinks at least 12 times in the prior year. Because older people have an increased sensitivity to the effects of alcohol and the common interaction with medications, you should pay particular attention to your alcohol consumption while you're taking medication.

Alcohol, when used in moderation, has a sunnier side. Many scientific studies now show that moderate drinkers live longer — longer than those who drink too much, and longer than those who don't drink at all. This is the case because alcohol affects the way that the body disposes of cholesterol. Drinking in moderation (two drinks a day for a man, one drink a day for a woman) is the key.

Cholesterol

Cholesterol is a good news/bad news story. It has been given a bad rap for all the problems associated with it, but we can't survive without it.

Cholesterol is a special kind of fat that serves mainly as a fat transporter. Cholesterol's principal function is to give rise to bile, an opaque green liquid stored in the gallbladder. Bile helps in the absorption of fat in the diet. When the gallbladder is informed by a chemical message sent by the stomach that some dietary fat is on the way down into the intestine, it squeezes a squirt of bile down its tube into the intestine where it mixes with the fat and facilitates its digestion. This is why fat in the diet gives rise to higher cholesterol levels. The liver is just doing what it is supposed to do.

Two-thirds of the cholesterol in the body comes not from the diet itself, but from the cholesterol that is manufactured in the body. The advice should be for a cholesterol-lowering diet, rather than a low cholesterol diet. Cholesterol in the food is a relatively minor contributor to the total body cholesterol. A cholesterol-lowering diet would mean lean portions of beef, lamb, or pork, no more than three times per week; low fat milk and cheeses; and no more than four eggs per week.

 Because cholesterol in food is a relatively minor part of body cholesterol, egg yolks are not as much a problem as often presumed. Four eggs per week is safe advice.

The cholesterol level in the blood responds to fat in the diet by the liver's manufacture. All dietary fats result in the liver producing more cholesterol, but unsaturated fats, the oils, compensate for this effect by helping in cholesterol's removal. This is the reason why animal fats are incriminated to a much higher degree than are their vegetable cousins.

But you must factor in the exercise element too. If a person eats a high fat meal but is physically active enough to burn the calories off, then it will not have the opportunity to settle into the sequence mentioned in the previous paragraph. Exercise is also helpful because of its partitioning property — it increases the good high-density cholesterol level (HDL). Whenever you check your blood cholesterol level, be sure that the HDL is included as well. When the HDL is high, as it is in most active people, total cholesterol is less problematic. For example, I would be more concerned if someone had 190 cholesterol with a 30 HDL than 210 and an HDL of 70. The total cholesterol/HDL ratio is the best indication of cholesterol safety.

People often say that, as you age, you get too old to worry about your cholesterol. This passive reassurance derives largely from the fact that experiments that have sought to lower cholesterol have not apparently lengthened the lives of the old dieters. People also point out that some older people are undernourished, and further restricting their dietary choices by a low-fat diet only serves to worsen this condition. I reject both these arguments. I feel strongly that it is never so late in life that you can stop being the best person you can be. If a 90-year-old enters my office and we find that his or her cholesterol is too high, I will offer advice about ways to get it down. The advice is probably nothing extreme, but it still holds true to the promise that, if life is worth living long, it is worth trying to live as healthfully as possible for as long as possible.

The role of drugs in the high cholesterol issue is still hotly debated. Good thinkers propose that vastly too much money is spent on medications to lower the cholesterol. I agree with this point. Drugs should always be the last recourse. Diet and exercise come at the top of the list, and drugs at the bottom. At the same time, however, in those people with high cholesterol levels who have already had a heart attack, or are suffering from angina, good solid evidence suggests that drugs can help diet and exercise lower the dangerous levels, and do save lives.

Getting Started: The Best Nutrition Plan for You!

Sample Weekly Menu for Week Beginning _____

	Monday	Tuesday	Wednesday	Thursday	Friday	Saturday	Sunday
Breakfast	Low-fat granola, yogurt, decaffeinated coffee or tea, juice	Scrambled eggs, dry wheat toast, fruit, decaffeinated coffee or tea, juice	Bagel with low-fat cream cheese, decaffeinated coffee or tea, juice	Low-fat cereal, fruit, decaffeinated coffee or tea, juice	Low-fat granola, yogurt, decaffeinated coffee or tea, juice	Pancakes, low-calorie syrup, lean breakfast meat such as turkey bacon	Low-fat blueberry muffins, fruit bowl, decaffeinated coffee or tea, juice
Lunch	Chef salad with skinless turkey and chicken breast, low-fat salad dressing	Tuna salad on whole wheat bread, pasta salad	Vegetable stir-fry, white rice, low-sodium soy sauce	Tomato basil soup, side salad with low-fat salad dressing	Grilled chicken sandwich, fresh cole slaw, fruit cup	Turkey burger patty, baked potato wedges, cup of minestrone soup	Turkey bacon/lettuce/tomato sandwich on whole wheat bread, bowl of fresh split pea soup
Snack	Fresh fruit	Frozen yogurt	Raw vegetables with low-fat dip	Frozen yogurt	Granola bar	Fresh fruit smoothie	Fresh salsa with low-sodium corn chips
Dinner	Grilled chicken breast, asparagus, roasted potatoes, small side salad w/ low-fat dressing	Pasta with red sauce, garlic bread, small side salad w/ low-fat dressing	Broiled white fish with lemon, baked potato, mixed vegetable medley	Beef tenderloin, steamed broccoli, brown rice	Roasted turkey breast, mashed potatoes, green beans	Turkey chili, cornbread, side salad w/ low-fat dressing	Grilled vegetable kabobs, brown rice, baked potato with salsa

Getting Started: The Best Nutrition Plan for You!

Weekly Menu for Week Beginning _____

	Monday	Tuesday	Wednesday	Thursday	Friday	Saturday	Sunday
Breakfast							
Lunch							
Snack							
Dinner							

Chapter 5

Getting Your R&R

• •

In This Chapter

▶ Sleeping enough

▶ Understanding why we all need to sleep

▶ Finding out how to get a good night's sleep

• •

*T*he third component of good health — after exercise and diet (which are covered in the preceding two chapters) — is rest. At first glance, rest would appear to be the easy part of staying healthy, but with the speed of life these days, rest is frequently the first thing people sacrifice. But cutting out an hour of sleep a night to get to work an hour earlier or running that last-minute errand before the store closes can harm your health over time.

People need to rest, absolutely. Sleep is just as critical to life as food and oxygen are. Studies show that animals that are kept awake artificially will die. If people are kept awake, they become disoriented and psychotic. I am not sure that anyone has ever died directly from lack of sleep, but many thousands have indirectly.

Getting eight hours of sleep a night is one of the most important determinants of how long people live. This observation was one of the key findings discovered in the famous Alameda County Study of long life conducted a few years ago. Sleep expert Dr. Bill Dement of Stanford, is convinced that insufficient sleep is the principal cause of some our recent major disasters such as Chernobyl, Three Mile Island, and the Exxon Valdez catastrophe, as the people at the controls were drowsy when they should have been alert. Beyond these headliners, however, are thousands of highway deaths due to "driving under the influence of sleep deprivation." But beyond even these direct causes, Dr. Dement feels that insufficient sleep is a substantial contributor to all sorts of other diseases, including heart disorders (which are worsened by erratic breathing patterns associated with poor sleep habits). I have never written "insufficient sleep" on any of the thousands of death certificates I have filled out. Maybe I should have.

Probably more important than the lethal effect too little sleep may provide, however, are the losses in good functioning that accompany a lack of sleep. Researchers have studied this aspect by progressively denying research volunteers one hour of sleep at night, then two, then four, and measuring the psychological and intellectual performances after each phase of withdrawal. Such studies show that mental capacities are highly correlated with the adequacy or inadequacy of sleep.

This chapter is devoted to down time — the time when we restore ourselves after running around like maniacs all day long. So sit back, relax, and enjoy the chapter!

The Need for Sleep and Relaxation

As Chapter 1 states, aging is the effect of energy on matter over time. The concept of how energy flow impacts matter is very important. If you have too much energy flow through matter, stress results. Too little energy, on the other hand, results in the disuse syndrome. (For more on the concept of aging, see Chapter 1). When too much or too little energy flow on matter lasts for some sustained period, then the organism becomes at risk.

Bob Sapolsky, professor of biology at Stanford, shows us that the reason zebras don't get ulcers (in fact, that is the title of his fine book) is because their challenges are intermittent with lots of down time in between. Presumably, if you could keep a zebra under a constant stress burden, it would develop ulcers, high blood pressure, and anxiety, as humans do. So, how we use our time, if we give ourselves time to wind down and relieve the stress and anxiety that is such a part of our daily lives, is key to how we age.

Sleep provides opportunity for repair needs and restores depleted supplies of crucial body chemicals. The eight-hour sleep allotment is related to our origins on the equator in Africa where the sun hides each night for eight hours. Cheating on millions years of sleep history is impossible.

The last several decades have revealed the sub-segments of sleep, meaning that brainwave studies differentiate parts of the sleep cycle, five different patterns including the rapid eye movement (REM) portion when most dreams and erections occur.

People in the United States are sleeping 20 percent less than they did 100 years ago. A person-in-the-street survey of residents of Los Angeles recently revealed that 32 percent of the respondents reported some degree of sleep difficulty. Fourteen percent reported a problem with falling asleep, 25 percent had trouble staying asleep, and 14 percent noted problems with early wakening. These figures are similar to others collected from all over the globe. So it seems we have a worldwide epidemic of insomnia going on.

The majority of insomniacs deal with the problem in a fairly casual manner. They do not generally contact physicians. Instead, people tend to self-prescribe relaxation techniques, physical exercise, reading, and over-the-counter medications as the preferred remedies. Twenty-eight percent of those surveyed on the streets of Los Angeles acknowledged using alcohol to help them get some shut-eye. Sleep problems are more frequently reported (69 percent) in those who do consult their physicians for whatever reason.

Losing downtime

Leisure time is evaporating. Pollster Lou Harris calculated that there has been a 37-percent reduction in leisure time in the United States in the last 20 years. Despite this fact, U.S. workers' productivity has doubled in the last 50 years! But instead of this productivity gain giving people freedom (by accomplishing more in less time), it has spawned the opposite problem. People are working longer, and more productively. U.S. employees put in 320 work hours more per year than their German and French counterparts. The Japanese are, if anything, worse off. The Japanese work 2,159 paid hours per year. People in the United States work 1,951 paid hours per year, compared to 1,614 in Germany and France.

The Wall Street Journal observed in 1996 that 40 percent of people feel that lack of time is a bigger problem than lack of money. Thirty-eight percent of people in the United States acknowledge "high stress." Fifty percent have high stress one to two times per week. Twenty percent note low stress. Those in professional and managerial casts are more crunched. Worker compensation claims for stress are way up. Stress rules the day, and with its predominance comes a cascade of negative health consequences, such as tension headaches, insomnia, and anxiety.

Take a lesson from me: I am not at all proud of how I have used my lifetime. One of my major regrets is the fact that I have difficulty shutting my eyes and remembering who our four wonderful kids were when they were 10 years old. In that era of my life, I was stringing together sequences of hundred-hour work weeks, tending a busy medical practice, and running a major research effort simultaneously. It was an orgy of self-gratification. In many ways, it was very productive in terms of good work, but I missed seeing my kids grow up. Thank goodness I had chosen a mate wisely, who more than compensated for my absent-dad syndrome. So I write this plea for good time management (check out *Time Management For Dummies,* 2nd Edition [Hungry Minds, Inc.], for tips on managing a busy life), more in the sense of do as I advise, not as I did. Fortunately, now in the grandchild era of life, I have matured and know how to allocate time more appropriately. Even if you are making the same mistake, you can stop now, hopefully sooner than I did, and start reallocating time more correctly.

It is calculated that over a lifetime we will spend six months in traffic, four years standing in line, and two years trying to connect on the telephone. Those hurry-up-and-wait experiences seem inevitable, but better planning can minimize wasteful minutes and hours.

Aging and sleep

Sleep complaints are heard often from older persons. A recent survey of 6,800 aging people in Boston, New Haven, and Iowa City, however, concluded that usually some non-related issue was the cause, rather than aging itself. Most common of these issues are medical conditions, often arthritis, which result in discomfort and adversely affects sleep patterns. Treatment of the underlying disorder is the correct approach to the sleep problem. This same study found that sleep disruption was generally short-lived. If aging was the cause, getting older would only make things worse. In addition to disease states, many medications are stimulating, which can cause sleep disruption. Many drugs used for heart or lung disease are stimulating. For example, cortisone and its derivatives are known stimulants.

Widely reported are changes in the anatomy of sleep as we age. The five levels of the sleep cycle get out of whack if we get less deep REM sleep. Further, the 24-hour natural cycle becomes shortened, resulting in the tendency to want to sleep at 6 p.m. and awakening at 3 a.m. ready to go. This situation, commonly called "sundowning," is seen in nursing home residents. Of course, the 3 p.m. to 11 p.m. staff shift is only too happy to let their charges hit the sack early. The 11 p.m. to 7 a.m. shift, however, confronts the group awakening at 3 a.m., ready to rise and shine. This setting has resulted in countless middle of the night phone calls to my home requesting a prescription for a sleeping pill — the correct approach, however, should be a rational rescheduling to prevent this phase shift.

Probably the biggest feature that impacts the sleep habits of older persons is physical inactivity. In a study supported by the American Association of Retired Persons, Doctors Abby King and Bill Haskell at Stanford found that prescribing physical exercise for a group of older persons who had complaints of insomnia resulted in a substantial reduction in sleep-related complaints.

So, once again, we face the issue of whether a problem said to be due to aging is in reality due instead to becoming inactive, and is thereby effectively helped by exercise. Exercise is cheap, safe, effective, and lacking in side effects. What sleeping pill can make that claim?

 The advice for an older person with a sleep problem are the same as those to a young person, except more so. Stay healthy, avoid medicines and stimulants, keep fit, stay on a schedule, and have a warm, quiet bed. Sleep tight.

Making Time for a Little R&R

Society's casual attitude toward diminished sleep is wrong. People need good sleep as much as they need exercise and good nutrition. Sleep is an integral part of the health triad. And this isn't just anecdotal information; in 1991, the National Sleep Foundation and the Gallup organization conducted a telephone survey of 1,000 randomly selected people in the United States. They asked questions about the ability to concentrate, capacity to tolerate annoyances, memory capacity, and irritability. Those with poor sleep habits showed a strong predisposition toward emotional and cognitive instability. Insomnia led to lower achievement, poorer health, job absenteeism, disability, and depression.

Cheating ourselves out of needed sleep

Knowing that sleep deprivation is bad, however, doesn't mean that we don't try to cheat. As a young doctor, I vividly recall pretending to be efficient the day after an all-nighter in the emergency room. I hope I didn't do too much harm, but such sleep-deprived performance loss has been the core issue in litigation about poor patient care. Stanford colleague and sleep expert Dr. Bill Dement points out that sleep deprivation is usually cumulative — an hour here, an hour there. The hours add up, and they must be paid back.

A good way of thinking about our absolute need for enough sleep is to imagine your functioning as a bank account that is deleted or credited by depositing or withdrawing one or two or ten nights of good sleep. It is possible to overspend for some brief period of time, but sooner or later the check (your functioning) will bounce as the result of overspending your sleep reserve. Unfortunately, there is only one way of repaying this debt and getting back into the black again — generating extra downtime.

Relax your cares away!

All things in nature delight in cycles. Acknowledging a downward dip in several body functions in the afternoon is nature's way of letting you know that some respite is needed to the clamor of the day. During my wife and my six-month sabbatical in Africa, we were repeatedly struck by how little was going on during the heat of the midday sun. Maybe there is a lesson there that our hurry up culture has forgotten — to our individual and collective peril.

Many scientific studies now attest to the many body and mind benefits that accompany downtime. The millions of adherents to meditation practice aren't wrong. Meditation lowers blood pressure, lowers stress hormones, improves digestion, lowers anxiety, improves sleep and memory, and allows freshness to emerge. During the quiet times, the two sides of my brain have a chance to talk with one another. The rest of the time, they are both so busy shouting that no communication goes on. Creativity emerges from the quiet times. Reflection is a health virtue with strong credentials.

Flow — that blissful state when all the gears mesh, when hard tasks become effortless, when time passes in an instant. We all need flow, but, in order for it to flourish, it needs the opportunity that simply cannot happen when life's sirens are all blaring at once. If someone were to ask me my definition of Hell, my quick response would be "a rock concert" — because to me these events are pure bedlam of no restorative value. Maybe I am growing old and crotchety, but please don't ever invite me to a rock concert.

Conversely, a good book, a massage, a long hot bath, a sunset, or an aquarium can be life extending. They give life its downtime. We all have need in ourselves for quiet places.

Getting a Good Night's Sleep

Millions of people have problems sleeping. Much of these problems are real, and many are imagined. My mother used to lament loudly about her inability to sleep, but sharing a bedroom on a trip certainly did not confirm this. Not infrequently, problem sleepers turn themselves into a sleep clinic for help. They are surprised and embarrassed to learn that despite their perception of their sleep pattern, when directly monitored, it is just fine.

So, the first issue to address is whether a person really has a sleep problem at all. Often an observer is necessary to confirm this supposed lack of sleep. If a real issue with poor sleep exists, it is important to ask whether any illness could be involved, including the following possibilities:

- ✔ Some hormonal conditions, such as an overactive thyroid gland, can cause sleep distress.

- ✔ Menopause often unsettles the rest pattern.

- ✔ The aches of arthritis are major sleep disrupters. Numerous therapeutic approaches are available that, when the distress is lessened, permit a good night's sleep.

- ✔ Both depression and anxiety are notable for their disruption of sleep.

- ✔ Many medications have stimulatory effects and must be acknowledged.

All of these concerns are the physician's responsibility to address. However, relatively few persons troubled by poor sleep turn to their doctors for assistance. Most of the time sleep disruptions are self-limiting and last only a few days. Patience is the cure for most insomnia. Said in another way, the body has a wonderful way of healing itself in many marvelous ways; among these ways is the body's tendency to reclaim sleep that has been lost without our conscious effort to redress it.

Triumphing over jet lag

Jet lag is evidence of how the body becomes distressed when its gears are not synchronized. Having flown over an ocean many times, I confess to the absurdity of pretending that nothing changes, and that the day of arrival can proceed normally at the new time setting. This strategy never works, and despite inconveniences and embarrassments, the sleep debit must be repaid before I can function again.

The two strategies that I have learned from the experts to help adjust my body's clock as quickly as possible after a jet trip are (1) exercise right away after the arrival, so that the activity cycle can be properly requeued, and (2) rehearse the arrival city's new time program a day or two before departing by resetting my watch and living in accordance with its schedule as much as possible before departure.

In addition to these two "tricks," I take melatonin. Melatonin is the body's sleeping pill. It is a natural substance made by the pineal gland in the brain and is the master coordinator of our circadian rhythms. Melatonin is widely available on the shelves of health food stores, but unfortunately, batches vary in their effectiveness. Possibly because of this uncertainty, scientists haven't yet found out the best use of the melatonin in jet lag situations. Melatonin's only side effect, so far as I know, is nightmares reported by some of its adherents. I am still experimenting, but there is a genuine promise that, after melatonin's use has been fully explored, we will all have hope for some respite from those grim, hung-over arrival mornings. If you are interested in melatonin, consult your physician before taking any.

Tips and tricks for falling asleep

You should have a routine before bedtime, so that your body can queue itself when the time comes to shut down. Going to bed at 8:30 p.m. one night, 1 a.m. the next, and 9 p.m. the next night messes up the body's signals. Environmental control is a basic and obvious helpmate for good sleep. Beds should be cozy, quiet, warm, and dark. Beds should be reserved for sleep time and making love, not for fretful ceiling staring. (Having a bedmate is associated with good sleep patterns.)

A lot of self-treatment of insomnia is common sense, so if you're having trouble sleeping, try these tips:

- Get rid of stimulants such as coffee, chocolate, tea, and nicotine. Your brain doesn't need chemical clamor as it winds down.

- Tend to your pet's and your own toilet needs before retiring. A full bladder is an alarm clock.

- Avoid heavy exercise before retiring. All the gears of the body and mind need to be in neutral for sleep to find a happy haven.

✔ Don't eat a big meal just before bedtime. A full belly means the body must attend to its needs and in so doing keeps the machinery going.

✔ Don't nap. A good night's sleep quota can be robbed by gratifying the rest need early in the day.

Avoiding sleeping aids

People in the United States love pills. Pills come in all shapes, sizes, and colors. Their uses span the imagination, so it's no surprise at all that sleeping pills are big. Fifty million prescriptions for sleeping pills and tranquilizers are written each year in the United States at a cost of over one billion dollars. And this doesn't include over-the-counter medicines! Enough sleeping pills are dispensed each year for every U.S. citizen to have a personal supply of 25 pills.

Sleeping pills are dangerous. They are addictive, and, in general, do much more harm than good. Of the hundreds of products available, none has been shown to be ideal. Some are short acting, and some are long acting. Hangovers are common. Sleeping pills disrupt the normal five-stage anatomy of sleep, and sleeping pills contribute to or aggravate depression. Their use with alcohol is particularly unwise. Regular sleeping pill users have a substantially higher mortality rate — in other words, sleeping pills shorten life. Sleeping pills are foreign chemicals for which the body is not prepared. None of the sleeping pills are smart enough to confer good sleep without demanding an unacceptable payback price. Don't pay the ransom demanded by taking a sleeping pill.

The only legitimate use of sleeping pills is to help reset the sleep clock to a normal routine after some disruption. This should take only a few days. Hopefully, melatonin (see the "Triumphing over jet lag" sidebar) will emerge as a safer and more effective tool for this purpose as well.

The best advice about sleeping pills: Don't take them!

Each of us, young, old, thin, chubby, rich, poor, and so forth, needs to make rest and relaxation a high priority. Not only does performance suffer without this dedication, but so too will length and quality of life. Plan on making rest as much a part of your health plan as diet and exercise! At the end of this chapter, you'll find a "Getting Started" worksheet sample along with a blank worksheet for you to develop your very own personalized relaxation plan. And we absolutely don't care if you photocopy the blank worksheet to reuse or share with friends!

Getting Started: Your Plan to Stay Rested and Ready-to-Go!

Sample Weekly R&R Plan for Week Beginning _____

	Monday	Tuesday	Wednesday	Thursday	Friday	Saturday	Sunday
Activity:	Reading/novel	Attending local community event (theater, concert, poetry reading, museum, festival, etc.)	Listening to music	Surfing the Internet	Reading/novel	Watching movie	Reading/magazine
Duration:	2 hours	3 hours	2 hours	2 hours	2 hours	2 hours	1 hour
Activity:		Coffee with friend		Writing letters, email			
Duration:		2 hours		1 hour			
Activity:	Afternoon nap	Afternoon nap	Afternoon nap	Afternoon nap			
Duration:	45 minutes	45 minutes	45 minutes	45 minutes			

Getting Started: Your Plan to Stay Rested and Ready-to-Go!

Weekly R&R Plan for Week Beginning _____

	Monday	Tuesday	Wednesday	Thursday	Friday	Saturday	Sunday
Activity:							
Duration:							
Activity:							
Duration:							
Activity:							
Duration:							

©2001 Hungry Minds, Inc.

Chapter 6

Using Alternative Medicine and Exercise Techniques

In This Chapter

▶ Yearning for something more than we have: the roots of alternative medicine

▶ Reaching for help from every source

▶ Putting "conventional" and "alternative" medicine together

*T*he name used to be "folk medicine." Then it was "holistic medicine," then "alternative," then "complementary," and now "integrative." And the word crafting isn't over yet! All of this effort has been spent out of a desire to differentiate nontraditional treatments from mainstream western medical practice. But if one-quarter of the world's population is currently using herbal remedies as the basis of therapeutics, and have been doing so for thousands of years, a person must ask: Which is the "conventional" medicine and which is "alternative"?

Lots of myths and many mysteries surround alternative medicine and exercise techniques. As with any treatment or routine, some alternative medicines are better than others, but in this chapter, I try to point out the pros and cons of some of the more popular methods. Communicating with your healthcare professional is a key component to living a longer, healthier life, and it is certainly important when considering alternative techniques. And if you hunger for more specific information than you find in this brief chapter, you can always turn to *Alternative Medicine For Dummies* (Hungry Minds, Inc.)!

Discovering the Difference: Conventional vs. Alternative

Western medicine is dominated by the use of drugs (see Chapter 18 and Appendix A for more discussion of medication). Scientific standards are used in their development to determine their usefulness, and they are only introduced to the market after a rigorous research developmental process.

The downside of medication, of course, is the high cost and potential side effects. Physicians rely heavily on the scientific underpinnings for the medicines we prescribe, validating through the double-blind testing technique in which neither the doctor nor the patient knows whether the test pill is the "real thing" or a dummy pill. This is the gold standard for usefulness and safety.

The lines between "traditional" and "alternative" medicine are anything but clear. Twenty years ago, I had the unpleasant responsibility of serving on a committee to look into the medical practice habits of one our hospital's staff. This fellow's medical practice was widely known to be very nontraditional. He said to me, "But Dr. Bortz, you can't sit in judgment on my practice because I, unlike you, am a holistic practitioner." "What's that?" I asked. "Why, I emphasize diet and exercise with my patients." Generally my temper is usually slow to rise, but this comment set me off. This man had maligned my like-minded colleagues and me by presuming that only he and his "holistic" colleagues considered the "whole" patient.

Unfortunately, conventional medicine and alternative medicine have gotten into a "them and us" scenario. The prevailing attitude is, "I'm right and you're wrong." With patients' health and a whole lot of healthcare dollars at stake, the argument has become heated.

My opinion of alternative vs. conventional medicine is hard-lined. I agree wholeheartedly with an editorial that appeared in the *New England Journal of Medicine* in September 1998, which stated that multiple scientific medicines do not exist, *there is only one*. There is no such thing as alternative or complementary or holistic medicine. There is only medicine.

Although I respect, accept, and encourage other ways of looking at medicine, I cannot endorse alternative medicine. I admit that much of traditional medicine remains unproven, and that the placebo effect exists (for more on that, see Appendix A). Still, my position remains that the scientific method, rather than testimonials, is the only standard of medical care.

I believe in the healing power of belief or faith — attitudinal healing is the affect of mind on body. Faith has positive effects on almost every human action. Faith works, and by verifiable scientific pathways. But, faith has its limits. A close friend of mine, Norman Cousins, brilliantly illustrates the power of positive thinking in his book *Anatomy of an Illness,* in which he explains the failings of medicine to deliver him from the pangs of serious illness, and how he only recovered when he assumed personal control of his illness. Norman's recovery led to his affiliation with UCLA School of Medicine as an adjunct professor, where he was devoted to attitudinal healing. In our relationship, I constantly tried to restrain his enthusiasm by noting the limitations of faith, while acknowledging faith's power. Norman was a good listener. His wonderful admonition, "Accept the diagnosis, reject the verdict," made room for both faith and hard reality.

The Budding of Alternative Medicine

The alternative medicine movement really took off in the 1960s, when the atmosphere of "challenge authority" ruled. People were dissatisfied with the status quo, and the medical establishment was a sitting duck for this rebellious spirit.

People believed that medicine's scientific growth was trampling over medicine's caring aspect. Some thought the patient was lost in the gadgetry and wizardry of technology, and machines had replaced the human touch. The specialist had replaced the family doctor. The emergency room had replaced the house call.

A romantic yearning for the good old days took hold of many people, and books on folk remedies sprung up, offering "nature's way of healing." This yearning was a backlash, and its appeal was obvious. By the 1980s, Senator Tom Harkin of Iowa was drafting legislation to include alternative medicine within the National Institutes on Health (NIH). In 1992, an office of alternative medicine was created within the NIH. The office's initial budget was $2 million a year and was rationed out to stimulate research.

The outcry from the medical establishment was loud and immediate. The new office was viewed as an acknowledgement of the validity of alternative medicine and a fundamental betrayal of trust. Despite this ongoing harping, the office's budget has risen to $68 million today, and its name has expanded to "The National Center for Complementary and Alternative Medicine." Although $68 million is still a pittance in comparison with the $15 billion total funding of the NIH, the amount of money going to this office is still increasing. Grudgingly, the establishment is making room for alternative medicine. Two-thirds of medical schools now offer classes about alternative medicine, and twelve university medical centers are funded by the NIH to pursue rigorous research projects on alternative ideas.

In some cases, being open to alternative medicine has yielded important clues. For example, a very aggressive form of childhood leukemia had been a mystery until researchers unlocked a key piece of evidence, which later was recognized as the same treatment that people had been using for 1,000 years in rural China, but without any understanding of why it worked.

Currently, over 15,000 papers concerning nontraditional remedies exist. Most research in these remedies is not designed properly (very little has used the double-blind technique, for example) and therefore is of sparse value. But change is coming.

The sad story of "miracle" cures

Much of the embrace of alternative medicine rests on testimonials of benefit or cure, some of which border on the miraculous, for restoration of long-lost capacities. They cater to deep yearnings for relief from serious problems from which conventional medicine has thus far failed. I predict an increasing fusion of traditional and nontraditional approaches, so that, before long, truly only one medicine will exist.

History shows we should be wary of alternative therapies reputed to produce miraculous effects. As recently as November 15, 1999, the *Journal of the American Cancer Society* reported a case of a "miracle" treatment in Italy. According to the article, recent tests of an anti-cancer therapy in use in Italy had been found to be almost completely ineffective. The treatment, created by Dr. Luigi DiBella from Modena, consisted of hormones, vitamins, and an anti-cancer medicine. The formula "MDB" was prescribed to all types of cancer patients, and Dr. DiBella claimed a cure rate of up to 100 percent, including improvement of patients who were terminally ill.

Because of the expense of the treatment, Italians wondered whether government insurance should pay for patients who could not afford it. The media got involved. Half of Italy's prime-time TV hours were devoted to the supposedly heavy-handed refusal of the National Health Service to supply this drug to anyone. The public demonstrated. The courts and the Pope got involved. Dr. DiBella's popularity grew as official medicine's fell.

In February 1998, the Italian parliament passed legislation that authorized a rigorous clinical trial of MDB's efficacy. Seven leading international cancer experts supervised this study. A total of 386 patients with cancer of all sorts were surveyed as to their response to MDB. Only three of the 386 cases showed any response. The results were made public in November 1998, and today, only a short time after that public furor, MDB has faded from the public imagination.

MDB is only one case in point. Fifty years ago in the United States, the drug laetrile was touted for cancer. The drug got robust support from several eminent scientists. The public, for its part, was eager for relief from the oppression of illness and had become critical of the tedious process required to develop legitimate treatments.

Why do such cases occur? Widespread distrust of the medical industrial complex, which sometimes creates conspiracy theories in which people believe that the establishment blocks drugs of potential value. I will tell everyone unequivocally: There is no process within the medical establishment that has an interest or action to prevent use of any drug or procedure of value. All concerned would meet any hint of such activity with immense scorn.

The lesson? The thousands of people who take these remedies of little or no value are forsaking traditional treatments, which, although far from ideal, are at least based on a rational approach. Don't replace experimental validation with faith. Anecdotes are insufficient reasons to embrace any therapy.

Yearning for something different

The alternative medicine movement (called "the new religion" by some) is the single fastest growing segment of healthcare. In 1990, 36 percent of people had seen an alternative medicine practitioner. By 1997, 47 percent had. Translated, this comes to 425 million visits to an alternative medicine practitioner in 1990 and 629 million in 1997. (This contrasts with the 386 million visits of persons to traditional practitioners in 1997.) In 1998, people spent $27 billion on alternative medicine.

The reassuring statistic is that only five percent of persons who visit alternative practitioners do so exclusively. The rest also see their regular physician.

If you are seeing an alternative medicine practitioner, let your doctor know. Many patients hide the fact that they are seeking "outside" help because they are embarrassed. Not telling your physician may be dangerous, because most alternative treatments can have side effects, which may be exaggerated if you are taking a standard prescription.

One survey indicated that 54 percent of the visits to alternative practitioners were to chiropractors, 25 percent to massage therapists, 14 percent to Chinese therapists (acupuncture, herbs, and so forth), and smaller percentages to other assorted healers. Health plans are wrestling with the consumer demand for these types of services, and more are including some allowance for use of these non-mainstream approaches. The largest number of health plan members request acupuncture (56 percent), while 45 percent seek chiropractic coverage, 25 percent seek massage, 21 percent seek biofeedback, and 8 percent seek coverage for hypnosis. The health plans of which I am aware vary greatly in the types of services that they allow, and the number of visits that they permit.

Sorting Between Good and Bad Therapies

The range of products, manipulations, and mental exercises of alternative medicine exceeds the imagination. Some common approaches, such as physical exercise, a sound diet, and relaxation skills do not belong in the alternative list at all — they are firmly in the category of standard medical practice. An abundance of firm scientific evidence documents their benefits.

Yet, alternative medicine has multiple recipes to offer, from mental visualization of cancer cells to rhino horn as an aphrodisiac, from electric current to prayer. Very few of these offer proven benefits, and some are outright dangerous. Most fall into the "may be helpful" category, however. When asked about the value of some nontraditional approach, my standard (and tedious!) answer is, "I don't know." If I have any prejudice in this answer whatsoever, it is a positive one, because I always look out for new approaches that may help patients. If physicians do not embrace every new remedy on first encounter, it is not because we are cynical or negative. The reason is because we have experience with poorly validated new products — medical history is littered with them. To help you avoid such products, this section gives you some insight into the most popular alternative medicine practices — the good and the bad.

Chiropractic practice

Chiropractic practice is the largest segment of the alternative medicine movement. Chiropractic is a form of healthcare that started in 1895, when Daniel Palmer, an all-purpose healer from Davenport, Iowa, coined the term *chiropractic* — the laying on of hands. The stated scientific rationale behind the chiropractic approach is the mal-alignment of the spinal vertebrae, which leads to problems with every body organ and system. People have claimed that the mal-alignment of dislocated vertebrae affects diseases as diverse as high blood pressure, bedwetting, immune function, asthma, and respiratory infections. The problem with the chiropractic proposition is that no substantial evidence verifies that these conditions are susceptible to spinal treatment. Further, traditional medicine still harbors major doubt that such a thing as dislocation of the vertebrae even exists, which throws the whole rationale of chiropractic into question.

A visit to a chiropractor's office usually involves taking a medical history, a physical examination emphasizing the spine, and an x-ray of the vertebrae. The chiropractor makes a diagnosis, and usually prescribes a series of readjustment sessions. Chiropractors cannot prescribe medication or perform surgery.

Most chiropractors confine their efforts to conditions of the musculoskeletal system, notably back pain. Evidence for the value of chiropractic treatment for back pain is meager, but it was enough for the federal agency for healthcare policy and research to state that chiropractic treatment was beneficial for acute low back pain.

Consistent evidence suggests that patients are pleased with their chiropractic experiences. Patient approval ratings for chiropractic are, in fact, higher than those of traditional medicine. This finding bothers me, but it doesn't surprise me. Chiropractors tend to spend more time with their patients than traditional practitioners do, and their service is generally much cheaper. Chiropractors act as health advocates. In addition, physicians' ability to address low back pain is poor, and made worse by the expense of our efforts. Customer service is a major element in medical care, and we traditionalists are doing a poor job of delivering patient-friendly service.

My hope is that the medical profession will learn about the art of health from chiropractors, and that the chiropractors will learn more about the science of health from us. The patient — who is the only person who really counts — will benefit from this exchange.

Osteopathy is occasionally confused with chiropractic. Osteopathy started with a focus on the musculoskeletal system as central to disease process. Gradually, however, osteopathy has become virtually identical to traditional medicine. Osteopaths do surgery and prescribe medicines. They can also be members of the American Medical Association.

Acupuncture

Despite thousands of years of use, acupuncture's principles remain obscure. This practice, derived from Chinese medical doctors, says that by inserting needles at selected specific points along the energy meridians — the hypothetical anatomic lines of connectivity — they can correct an imbalance in the flow of *qi* (pronounced like "key"), the vital life energy. An imbalance of qi is considered the cause of disease.

There may well be some truth to the principle of qi, as several studies indicate a discernable physical basis for the meridians of Chinese medicine. Still, no definitive proof exists, and we await further scientific insights.

Acupuncture's principal use is for pain relief, major university medical centers list acupuncture among their treatments in their pain clinic protocols, and insurance companies pay for it, so some validation is at hand. Other reported conditions for which acupuncture is of value, such as hypertension, infertility, and anxiety, are still in the "don't know" column.

Magnet therapy is a cousin of acupuncture. The principle is to use magnets instead of needles. Like acupuncture, much skepticism surrounds the claims of magnet therapy, but two recent research efforts on diabetic- and shingles-associated pain seem to affirm its benefit for pain relief. We'll see.

Body-mind medicine

Body-mind medicine is a no-brainer. Of course the mind, the attitude, and the spirit participate in keeping a body whole! By adhering to this practice, you get the best of both worlds — a concentration in muscular strength, aerobic levels, flexibility, and balance with a mental focus that's both inward-focused (on the body) and contemplative (on the mind). Yoga, pilates, and Tai Chi are examples of popular mind-body fitness activities. (For more information on how you can incorporate yoga and pilates into your workout, see *Weight Training For Dummies,* 2nd edition [Hungry Minds, Inc.].) In my opinion, body-mind medicine contains nothing alternative, but the skepticism from many surrounding the body-mind connection has pushed it into the realm of alternative medicine.

Pessimists get sick, optimists stay well. That's nature's way. Not all pessimists get sick, however, nor do all optimists stay well. Body-mind medicine is not an all or none connection. And, sometimes the best medical solution is a simple physical solution. If I get a thumbtack in my foot, the correct response is not psychotherapy, or prayer, or transcendental meditation, but to take the thumbtack out! Likewise, if a patient has a breast lump, the first response should be surgery or other direct therapy rather than joining a support group. Conversely, if a person is beyond the limits of standard medical assistance, the best treatment is not more chemotherapy, but steps that provide love, comfort, and dignity.

For more specific information, pick up a copy of *Mind-Body Fitness For Dummies* (Hungry Minds, Inc.)!

Supplements: Herbs and vitamins

In the realm of supplements — material in addition to the standard table fare — alternative medicine espouses that if some is good, more must be better. Getting your nutrients is perfectly correct: Sound science teaches that our well-being depends on a proper mixture as specified by the food pyramid (see Chapter 4), just as a car needs good gas and oil to function.

Nutritional supplements are a growth industry. Thirty to fifty percent of people in the United States take some supplement. Six hundred suppliers provide four thousand products! No one can keep up with the vast array of products, and consumers spend billions of dollars in the pursuit of something, which will gain that extra boost or give that edge in stamina, sexuality, or beauty.

A few supplements have documented value. Calcium, folate, fiber, and restricted sugar consumption are definitely valuable. Other substances are of unlikely value. Shark cartilage, touted as a cancer treatment

because sharks don't get cancer, is one example. Super oxide dismu-
tase, chromium, selenium, and co-enzyme Q produce millions of dollars
for their manufacturers, but have almost no proven value. In addition,
the purity of these supplements is highly questionable. In 1998, the
California Department of Health checked out 260 herbal remedies and
found that other substances contaminated one-third of the remedies.

Herbs, too, are widely used as supplements and remedies. Many have
potent ingredients in their formulation. Some can be dangerous. A widespread conviction exists that states if a pill is of "natural" origin, it must
be totally safe. Wrong! Some herbs can kill when used inappropriately.

The supplement industry's main problem is lack of regulation. Herbs,
such as Gingko, Echinacea, or ephedra, are not required to document
either effectiveness or danger to the same degree that a new blood
pressure medicine or hormone preparation is. Consequently, taking
these products comes down to the old caution, "Buyer beware!"

Some supplements work, while others might work. Critical efforts are
underway to assess what effects, good and bad, these compounds are
having when they are subjected to a rigorous analysis. In the meantime,
here is what we know scientifically about popularly used supplements:

Ginseng

The word *ginseng* comes from a Chinese word for "likeness of man." (In
China, roots that resemble the human form are particularly valued.)
Ginseng's proper name is panax, which comes from the Greek word
panacea, meaning "all-healing." And, indeed, ginseng is a Chinese cure-
all. Ginseng's use is believed to set everything right with the world.
Medicinally, the root is considered valuable by alternative practitioners for treating fevers, inflammation, and hemorrhage and pain of childbirth. Some people claim that Ginseng's use promotes vigor and sexual
desire. I know of no medical experiments that validate ginseng's value.

Gingko biloba

This product, derived from the gingko tree, is reputed to have positive
effects on the central nervous system. A fair amount of research has
focused on gingko biloba's use. An article in the October 1998 issue of
the *Journal of the American Medical Association* found a modest benefit
in mental acuity when given to persons with Alzheimer's disease.
Gingko biloba's effect on other nervous system-related disorders, such
as Parkinson's disease, failing memory, or stroke, is unclear, pending
further research.

Saw palmetto

This product, widely heralded for prostate health, does indeed work —
but at a price. Saw palmetto is an identified source of plant estrogens
that act to shrink the prostate gland. This is very useful, as many older

men suffer a condition known as benign prostatic hypertrophy, meaning that the prostate gland swells. (When the prostate gets bigger, it interferes with urinary function, causing many middle-of-the-night trips to the toilet. This condition is very common and very annoying.) Saw palmetto works because the prostate is a hormonally sensitive organ and is stimulated by the male hormone testosterone and inhibited by the female hormone estrogen. The bad news about saw palmetto is that estrogen-like effects obscure the value of the prostate specific antigen test, a very important blood test for prostate cancer. PSA is our best indication of the early presence of prostate cancer, and I, for one, would never confound the accuracy of a PSA test by taking saw palmetto.

Echinacea

Echinacea is the biggest selling herbal remedy and is used to alleviate the common cold, flu, and respiratory infection. Echinacea is said to enhance immune responsiveness. Although a few studies do indicate its usefulness, the studies are of marginal quality. More research is needed.

Saint John's Wort

Saint John's Wort is promoted for treating depression and is used widely in Europe. In Germany, more people use Saint John's Wort than Prozac and other standard antidepressant medications. A report in the *British Medical Journal* found that Saint John's Wort worked about as well as antidepressant medications. Hypericum perforatum (the proper name for Saint John's Wort) has been used since ancient Greek times. While Saint John's Wort certainly contains active ingredients, we need to find out what they are and how to use them wisely. One warning: A recent article in the leading British medical journal, the *Lancet,* found that people who are taking Saint John's Wort are at risk if they are compromised by treatment for AIDS or for organ transplants.

Melatonin

Melatonin is a natural product, made in the brain's pineal gland, just as cortisol, thyroxin, and estrogen are. Melatonin's purpose is to synchronize daily rhythms and has been marketed to health food stores by the bushels. The trouble is that melatonin's production is not standardized, and we haven't figured out yet how to use it. After it is standardized, Melatonin should prove especially effective for jet lag or night shift difficulties by helping to reset our inner clocks more efficiently. So far, melatonin hasn't shown to have any adverse effects other than nightmares in some people.

Vitamins

When taking vitamins, many people seem to think that if a little is good, more must be better. Wrong. Several vitamins, if taken in excess, can be hazardous. The health benefits of a balanced diet including fruits, vegetables, and grains are a sure thing, but taking a handful of vitamins does not replace eating a balanced diet. A good food program has dozens of other micronutrients that you can't get from a synthetic diet of vitamin pills.

People who eat a good diet have a lower incidence of cancer. No nutritional vitamin supplement can make that claim. The message? Eat well. If, for whatever reason — dental, economic, social — you are not eating according to the food pyramid recommendations, add a supplementary multivitamin to your daily regimen.

Supplements can have adverse effects when combined with prescribed medications. Always tell your physician what over-the-counter medicines you are taking.

This short list of remedies is not intended to be comprehensive. For those who are interested in the whole gamut of alternative alternatives, such as chelation, copper bracelets, and aromatherapy, numerous reference sources abound. A favorite one is "The Best Alternative Medicine — What Works? And What Does Not?" written by Stanford colleague Ken Peletier. Also, be sure to check out *Alternative Medicine For Dummies* (Hungry Minds, Inc.).

Choosing Alternatives Wisely

Human nature compels us to try to find better and easier ways for everything. This rejection of the status quo can serve us well, but we must always ask whether the new device is better than the old choice, even if the old choice is imperfect.

Efforts to influence society's drug use pattern now involve slick campaigns that feature your favorite sports figure, politician, or TV personality giving their earnest testimonials about such-and-such a salvation product. Buyer beware! Whenever anything or anyone presumes that this service or that supplement can cure or alleviate baldness, shortness of breath, sexual inadequacy, diabetes, achy joints, and a dozen other afflictions, back off. A hundred Nobel prizes await such a product, and that recipient has yet to be found.

The proper stance of any older person (myself and my wife included) is to be aware, curious, and free to ask questions. Cynicism is inappropriate, but healthy skepticism isn't. We should all want to know the latest information about all new products, traditional and nontraditional. It is our responsibility not to adopt a negative attitude about anything new or out of the ordinary because no one has the final, ultimate insight into what is right for us, except us.

Alternative medicine doesn't exist. In my opinion, only the right medicine for us exists — conventional medicine and alternative medicine is all the same thing.

Hitting the Mat: Meditation, Yoga, and Other Alternative Exercise Techniques

Alternative medicine isn't the only way to supplement your physical and mental health. Alternative exercise techniques include several practices that focus on both physical and mental well-being.

Meditation involves a variety of mental and physical techniques that show you how to relate to different circumstances in your life. With focused mental introspection and breathing and stretching patterns, you learn how to balance everything life throws at you. Meditation can help you handle anxiety, stress, loneliness, isolation, depression, and stress-related illness.

Yoga includes exercises that look a lot like gymnastics. These exercises can help you stay fit, lose weight, develop better flexibility, and relieve stress. Yoga also combines many meditation practices with these exercises that exercise your lungs and calm your nervous system. Many people find yoga incredibly invigorating and energizing!

Other similar exercise methods include pilates, Tai Chi, and power yoga (a more aerobically charged version of yoga).

For more detailed information, grab copies of *Meditation For Dummies, Yoga For Dummies,* and *Mind-Body Fitness For Dummies* (all published by Hungry Minds, Inc.).

Part II
The Psychological Aspects of Living Longer

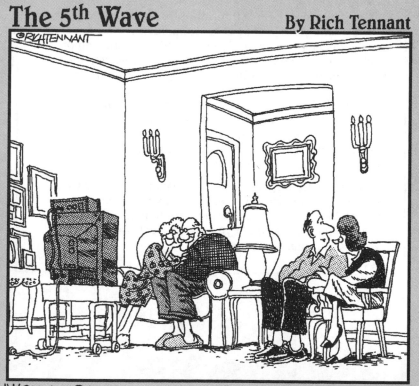

The 5th Wave   By Rich Tennant

"MOM AND DAD GET LIKE THIS EVERY TIME THEY WATCH BACK-TO-BACK EPISODES OF 'THE LOVE BOAT.'"

In this part . . .

When most people think about working out, weight lifting and jogging come to mind. But, you can't neglect giving your *brain* a workout. It's the most important organ you've got. Remaining an active participant in life is one of the best ways to prolong your life. Check out Chapter 7 for some great tips on keeping your brain active. Working is definitely one way to keep your brain in shape, but once retirement comes, does that mean your chances for keeping your brain sharp are diminished? Certainly not! Look to Chapter 8 for guidance on how to keep your brain fit after you retire.

Worries about keeping sexually active and deciding where to live out your last years can certainly create strain on the brain. Chapters 9 and 10 are here to help alleviate your concerns and to put you on the right track for balancing your life.

Chapter 7

Maintaining Your Brain Power and Engaging in Life "Sense-ibly"

. . . .

In This Chapter

▶ Keeping in touch with the world through your senses

▶ Understanding that aging doesn't diminish the senses

▶ Monitoring your vision, hearing, and ability to smell and taste

▶ Staying creative to stimulate your senses

. . . .

Staying in touch with family and friends, engaging your mind and body in challenging ways, and participating in a variety of activities are central strategies for a successful aging. The richness of your personal involvement with other people is key to having a good quality of life. Being alone and out of touch just doesn't cut it. Maintaining contact with the outside world is a survival tool as necessary as eating and breathing.

This necessity is apparent at every level of our beings — from the cellular level, to the personal level, and up to the community level. Cells derive their shape and function from their peripheries. When you touch somebody, that energy is transmitted by the nerves to the spinal cord and then to the brain where it is perceived. This energy chain actually changes the nerve and brain anatomy, like a muscle builder's biceps in response to chin-ups. In a real way, people become what they do — touching and sensing is a big part of living. At the personal level, as Barbra Streisand sang, "People who need people." At the community level, the notion of one world, the global village, unifies us all to a more complete existence. Stimulating your senses through creativity will also keep you sharper. Listening to music, writing, reading, watching movies, going to the theater, and other activities will help keep you engaged and on top of the world!

Interacting with Others Through Our Senses

Interaction is a fact of life. In fact, interaction *is* life. A mountain of evidence asserts that the more acutely you maintain your interactive capacities, the more your days will gratify you. Our senses — hearing, seeing, tasting, touch (balance), smelling — enable us to interact with others. Sensitivity to temperature is another sense that older people need to be aware of. While many animals possess specific sensory capacities keener than our own, and even totally different than our own (bats and their night "radar" come to mind), there is no question that human beings are richly endowed with magnificent antennae that tune us in to our world.

Human beings have been called the most adaptable of all species, and certainly we have an unsurpassed ability to experience and react to an immense array of surroundings. The earliest life-forms detected their environment only by bumping into it. Progressive development facilitated sensory capacities at a distance. Sensing means capturing a particular kind of energy, light, or heat, or pressure, or acid. This energy is caught, recognized, and analyzed to inform and instruct the body as to how to react to its environment.

Not being able to use our senses is torture. Sensory deprivation, in which persons are confined to near-zero environmental contact, has been widely exploited as a torture and brainwashing device. Loss of contact with meaningful surroundings quickly leads to disorientation and hallucinations. Even a short-term loss of contact means deterioration in our senses. For example, when you wake up and get out of bed after a long night's sleep, your sense of balance may be slightly off due to your visual and equilibrium senses being dulled by sleep.

Denying ourselves the opportunity to use our sensing apparatus is a bad, bad thing, but what about the reverse? Can we train the senses to be better than average? Can we see, hear, or smell more acutely if we practice? Can a blind person hear better than a sighted person, for example? Can a deaf person see more?

The answer to these questions is similar to the answers to questions about increasing our intelligence. Decreasing a person's intelligence by impoverishing his or her environment is easier than increasing a person's intelligence by enriching the environment. By the same token, decreasing your sensory perception by not exercising your senses is easier than heightening your senses by exposing yourself to more sensory input. I'm not saying that improving your senses is impossible, mind you. More and more information is emerging about the moldable nature of our nervous system, and the sensory organs are part of the nervous system. Some evidence suggests that you can work to sharpen certain senses. For example, musicians seem to hear differently from the rest of us. The ability called *perfect pitch* — being able to hum or whistle a particular note, such as middle C, on demand — is rare, but is much more common in people who had intense exposure to music early in life.

Taking Hold of Your Senses as You Age

Sensory capacities help determine our quality of life at any age — but particularly as we grow older. A recent survey of 576 older persons with an average age of 78 indicated that 18 percent had impaired vision and 64 percent had diminished hearing. Compared to a perfect score of 20, which indicates full functioning in all the day's activities, those persons with no sensory loss scored 14, indicating mild impairment in getting through the day. Those with hearing loss alone scored 11, those with visual loss alone scored 10, those with both hearing and visual loss scored 8. These lower values place these persons with lesser function and diminished life quality at risk of needing nursing home care. The authors of that study concluded that while sensory loss may not be thought of as catastrophic, it may well represent the difference in being able to remain at home and needing to go to a nursing home.

The senses generate independence. Loss or diminishment of our senses generates dependency. In fact, loss of vision and balance clearly increase one's likelihood of falling, and falling can be fatal, either directly or indirectly.

Too often, people have passively assigned losses in vision, hearing, taste, smell, and balance to aging itself. Doctors have a term for two types of sensory loss blamed on age: *presbyopia,* for vision loss, and *presbycusis,* for hearing loss (*presby* is a prefix meaning *old*). Both terms imply that age causes the sensory loss. But what if diminished vision or hearing or smell or taste or balance is not "presby" in its origin, but rather something that needs reclassifying?

"Presby" implies that you can't do anything about a problem — that you have to, as the Serenity Prayer states, "accept what you must." But "change what you can" is the more appropriate and helpful strategy to take care of your senses.

I feel strongly that taking care of your senses is one of the most important — and most neglected — ways to live long and well. If we paid as much attention to our senses as we do to our teeth and to our hairstyles, we would all be a lot better off. Not that teeth and hair aren't important, but in the hierarchy of importance, seeing and hearing, for example, are much more significant!

Our collective neglect of our senses is an example of Zimmerman's Law in operation: Nobody notices when everything is okay. Studies show that not until 70 percent of our sensory capacity is lost do we start to become concerned that there may be a problem. But even then, many people do not react promptly to address their deficit. Millions of people who need and can clearly benefit from easily available help don't make the first phone call. Why? Many of them are in denial. People don't like to wear glasses or hearing aids. They believe the need for a hearing aid, for example, is an acknowledgement of aging and decline, which is something that happens only to the other guy or gal. But what if the cause isn't aging? What if there is something you can do to improve the situation?

You must tend to your senses as you age. Honor them, value them, protect them, test them, repair them, and be aware of them. If you have a problem, get a diagnosis, and know what you must accept and what you can change.

The basic framework for knowing what to accept and what to change (see Chapter 1) works for the senses too. Genes, injury, poor maintenance, and aging are the four categories that can cause loss of sensing. As we age, genetic conditions are minimal as contributors, so you can dismiss that category. Aging is a possible cause of diminished sight, hearing, and so forth, but because we can't do anything about aging, we will acknowledge it as a contributor, and then move on. Injury and maintenance, however, can contribute to late-life sensory loss. But before we accept aging, per se, as the cause of sensory loss, we need medical advice to be sure that injury and poor maintenance are not involved because the good news is that you can remedy sensory loss caused by injury and maintenance.

Increasing evidence suggests that cumulative damage from sunlight or noise is a major contributor to vision and hearing deficits. Balance, too, is affected by the disuse subsequent to diminished cueing of the equilibrium apparatus. Inattention to balance unquestionably hastens its deterioration and, importantly, can be offset by a simple intervention strategy. The balance intervention strategy is the flamingo stand described in the Chapter 3. It seems unlikely that vision and hearing are compromised by underuse because we seem to have them in constant awareness, but you can implement specific eye exercises that are designed to curtail loss of distance accommodation. A substantial portion of the losses that have previously been passively accepted as inevitable parts of aging now lend themselves to a preventive or corrective strategy. How can we maintain the senses of sight, hearing, smell, and taste, as well as balance and temperature, as we age?

Keeping an eye on your vision

Loss of vision is the most dreaded of the sensory deficits and is a common affliction, with 29 percent of a group of 1,200 centenarians surveyed professing some vision loss. Of the 1,200, 49 (4 percent) were blind, 37 (3 percent) reported cataracts, and four (.3 percent) had glaucoma. On the bright side, 104 (9 percent) didn't use glasses at all. Among the group was one person who had a cataract removed at age 99, and another who gained back lost vision with surgery for cataract disease.

Other studies have shown that on average, 11 percent of people over 65 years of age report some functional visual impairment. This figure rises to 21 percent in the 75 to 85 year age group, and 42 percent in those over 85. The average age at which reading glasses become necessary is 45.

The list of things that can adversely affect the eyes is substantial, and, luckily, the majority of them can be managed if diagnosed in time. I strongly encourage routine eye doctor visits for everyone over 60 years of age. By adopting a routine exam program, your doctor can note any loss of vision. Sudden vision changes, pain in the eye, flashing lights, or double vision should prompt an immediate visit. Eyesight is so precious that procrastination and denial make no sense whatsoever!

I am delighted to be able to add yet another item to the list of benefits of physical exercise. When both sight and hearing are tracked in groups of fit and unfit persons, those people who are in better condition also demonstrate superior eyesight and hearing. I guess this information should be predictable because of the global benefits of exercise, but I am always on the look out for ways to negate or alleviate negative aspects of growing older. If something as simple, safe, and cheap as an exercise program can offset even a small part of the sensory losses of aging, then you have even one more reason to exercise.

Avoiding cataracts

A cataract is the familiar greyish clouding of the lens of the eye. Two-thirds of visual problems are a result of alterations in the shape, elasticity, and clarity of the eye's lens, leading to distorted, fuzzy images. Of these lens changes, half are due to cataract formation. Careful eye checks reveal that half of all people begin some cataract formation before age 65.

People with cataracts see the world as though their eyes have petroleum jelly smeared on them. Their vision is dim and fuzzy. One million cataract operations are performed each year, amounting to one of the largest Medicare expense items (12 percent of Medicare's total expenses). This simple operation consists of removing the clouded lens of your eye and replacing it with a plastic one that is balanced with the lens of the other unoperated eye. Hundreds of my patients have undergone this operation, and their acclaim for its results is nearly universal.

No one is quite sure what causes cataracts. People have proposed smoking, diabetes, and cortisone as possible causes, but ultraviolet light exposure is the leading suspect. A study of Chesapeake Bay fishermen established a dose-effect relationship: Those who spent the most time squinting at the bright sun had the highest incidence of cataract disease. Snow reflection is also known to be harmful to your eyes.

Currently, the National Institutes of Health is sponsoring a number of research projects to see whether vitamins, zinc, or antioxidants protect against the development of cataracts. Green vegetables are widely touted as anti-cataract agents. In addition keeping the blood sugar under control if you have diabetes is a substantial proven preventive strategy for cataracts.

Managing macular degeneration and glaucoma

Only about 9 percent of older people develop *macular degeneration,* which causes a blind spot at the point of concentrated vision. Macular degeneration is a substantial burden, but, fortunately, it never results in total blindness. Encouraging new attempts at therapy involve growth function and laser use.

Glaucoma, which is characterized by increased pressure with the eye causing impaired vision and may lead to total vision loss, affects 11.5 million persons. Eye drops can usually manage this condition.

Older persons also commonly note *floaters* — tiny squiggles that drift across their vision. These result from fragments of collagen breaking off into the fluid of the eye. They are related to actual tears in the retina, which are immediately suspected if vivid flashing lights are seen in the periphery of the visual field. Flashing lights are an alarm signal to call the eye doctor because emergency treatment can prevent further damage.

Lending an ear to your hearing

Deafness or partial hearing loss is a profound issue in millions of older persons, and many older persons deny that they even have this problem. Estimates claim that 70 percent of persons who can benefit from a hearing aid don't get around to getting one. This is a great sadness because the problem is so widespread. I recall attending a medical meeting in Boston and hearing a lecture entitled "Demented, depressed, or deaf?" It was a provocative title, but an apt one, because it alerted us physicians to the masquerade that loss of hearing often presents.

In the centenarian study cited earlier in this chapter in the vision section, about 26 percent of the subjects reported substantial deafness, which, they commented, was less worrisome than their visual defects. Other surveys report higher incidences. Tom Perls, who is the director of the Harvard Centenarian Study, reports that 30 percent of persons over 65 have diminished hearing — that's 9.4 million of us. This hearing loss leads to a succession of psychological frustration and withdrawal. Social ties loosen, and depression and even dementia are threats. As an example, many people with hearing loss report that they stop attending religious services because they can't hear the sermon.

Most experts now agree that people could avoid most hearing loss if they weren't exposed to loud noises. Noise-induced hearing loss is very common. In fact, I ran across an interesting article regarding hearing tests conducted on a group of natives of an isolated Pacific island, Easter Island. Their hearing was magnificent until they went to work abroad. Upon retesting (after six months), they were found to have lost substantial amounts of their previously keen hearing ability. No hearing loss is noted in primitive tribes, but 60 percent of college freshmen in the United States already have evidence of diminished hearing. During my six-month sabbatical in Africa, I spent as much time as I could away from urban areas. The quiet out there startled me. That's the way our ancestors evolved, in the quiet — totally different than the clamor of New York City, where even the wee hours of the night are ripe with assaults on the eardrum.

Loudness is measured in *decibels*. Normal conversation is at the 40-decibel level, a dog bark is 80, a telephone ring 90, and power tools and rock concerts are 100. A firecracker or gunshot is 170 decibels. One gunshot is equivalent to one week of occupational noise. It's not just the intensity of the noise that counts, duration does as well.

Although some very acute losses of hearing may be temporary, most injuries caused by noise tend to be cumulative and lead to an old age with diminished hearing. One loud bang equals scar tissue in the tender ears. Two loud bangs equal two scars, and on and on until your ears are too scarred to work properly. Avoiding sounds over 75 decibels is a good idea. Ear plugs and protectors are sound preventive medicine.

Hearing loss tends to occur first in the high part of our hearing range. Some conversational tones, "f" and "s" for example, exist more in the high ranges. The vowels tend to occupy the lower frequencies. A person with a selective high-tone loss will hear incomplete sentences or words with specific sounds missing.

The ear tissues are not exempted from drying, atrophy, and loss of elasticity, conditions over which you have little control. Because excessive noise has the largest role in provoking deafness, however, you should change what you can by avoiding exposure to loud noise. (Also don't forget to keep your ear clear of wax. Unquestionably, many older persons are suffering the indignity of hearing loss merely because their ears are full of wax, which is easily and conveniently cleaned out.)

Simple soapy water with a rubber syringe is usually all that is necessary to keep ears clean. If this doesn't work, there are a number of ear drops (Cerumenex or Debrox) that are stronger. If these fail, your doctor's nurse is probably an expert at ear wax removal.

Sometimes deafness is associated with ringing in the ears — *tinnitus* is the medical word. Thirty percent of people over 55 years of age have mild ringing, and in 10 percent of those people the ringing may be severe. High blood pressure, stress, aspirin, caffeine, and a list of other medications can provoke buzzing noises, which are sometimes very troublesome. These noises are often hard to treat, and you should consult an audiologist for medical assessment and treatment.

If you have a hearing problem, try to avoid the kind of *competing noise* that is so often found in places like busy restaurants, such as air conditioners, traffic, or dish clatter. Keep conversation simple, slow, and direct, and don't shout. Use writing and other cues when appropriate. You may also need a hearing aid, which you can determine by a visit to your friendly audiologist. I recommend a baseline visit at age 60 for everyone and then every five years thereafter, unless symptoms intervene and a sooner visit is appropriate.

Doctors prescribe two million hearing aids each year in the United States, although only a small percentage of those hearing aids are worn — and that's too bad. The good news is that the effectiveness of various aids is vastly improved. For those persons in need of an aid but unable to afford one, Hear Now (9745 E. Hampden Ave., #300, Denver, Colorado 80231), may provide one free or at reduced cost. Certainly recovery of lost hearing should be worth a good investment.

Checking your balance

Because balance is another sense that resides partially in the ear anatomy, its loss often follows the departure of hearing. Balance is a multi-organ function, which involves the brain, eyes, spinal column, muscles, peripheral position sense recorders, and the inner ear (where our "gyroscope" resides within the semicircular canals). When this complex system is working, we maintain our equilibrium under all sorts of upsetting circumstances, but when any part of the system is defective we become at risk of a fall.

As with seeing and hearing, most of us take balance for granted. A fall often precipitates the first recognition of the problem. Certainly age plays a role in decreased balance. For example, our capacity to detect vibration goes down with aging. Still, much evidence indicates that you can improve your balance by simple exercises such as the flamingo stand (see Chapter 3 for more information on balance exercises).

A particularly troubling kind of imbalance is vertigo. Vertigo is the severe form of dizziness in which the room or you actually seem to be spinning. Substantial numbers of older people suffer from serious vertigo. We have learned now that a large portion of these persons suffers from the development of little crystals within their semicircular canals of the inner ear. Change in position of the head causes these crystals to brush against the sensing hairs in the canals and convey the sensation of dizziness. Certain head-positioning exercises — available at your doctor's office or from an ENT specialist — can be done to encourage the crystals to "settle out" and thereby hinder their irritative effects.

If you have vertigo or any other difficulties with your balance, consult your doctor for a referral to an otolaryngologist who specializes in balance disorders.

Monitoring your senses of smell and taste

We don't know very much in detail about the senses of smell and taste and how they change when we age. We know there are 1,000 different smell-detecting proteins in the nose, leading to the great precision of our sniffing apparatus. Both the intensity and the differentiating capacity to smell diminish with the years. The same holds true for taste; we may find certain foods too bitter at a young age and then able to handle them as we age. This phenomenon leads many older people to seek more flavor in their food. Gourmets and professional perfume sniffers claim not to suffer such losses, but whether "use it or lose it" applies to these senses as well is simply unknown.

Smoking is bad for taste and smelling capacity, as it is for everything else.

If your ability to smell and taste declines significantly, you may ultimately experience decreased pleasures of eating. If you believe your senses of taste and smell are diminished, have your doctor consider dental and medication issues. Sometimes dental fillings or gum infections may alter taste. A long list of drugs can provoke senses of bitterness or acid or metal.

Watching the thermostat

Newspapers regularly announce increased deaths of older people during particularly cold or hot weather spells. In 1990, 9,000 people in the United States died of hypothermia. Your risk of dying of hypothermia doubles if you are over age 65, and increases to five times the average if you are over 75. On average, 300 people die each year from overheating. The scorching heat of 1980 caused 1,700 deaths — 80 percent of which occurred in people over 50.

Extremes of temperature affect older people because their heat and cold sensing capacities — their inner thermostats — are diminished. The brain contains centers that control both sweating and shivering. Experiments have clearly shown that older people require more disruption of the environmental temperature before accommodating reactions set in. Insulation issues are also a factor. Many older people, particularly the frail, lack subcutaneous fat that serves to buffer the cold. Other older persons with excess fat are, in effect, surrounded by a heat blanket, which places them at increased risk for overheating.

The basal metabolism, which is dependent on lean body mass, generates most of the body heat. As older persons lose muscle mass, their heat production decreases. In addition, disease states, such as vascular problems; central nervous system diseases, such as Parkinson's disease; infection; or kidney failure also diminish our temperature control capacity by disrupting the complex thermoregulatory reflexes.

Alcohol is an additional demon in the impact of temperature extremes on older individuals. Alcohol not only numbs the senses, but also adversely redistributes the blood so that heat loss in increased.

With all these precautions about avoidance of temperature extremes, older persons are capable of accommodating to altered temperature habits — just make sure to use common sense and vigilance. Listen to the weather reports, and if a heat wave or cold spell is in your neighborhood, stay indoors. Set your thermostat or air conditioner at a comfortable level.

Keeping Your Windows to the World Wide Open

Don't take your senses for granted. Guard them, recognize if they are suffering in the least, and cherish them. Don't assume that any lessening of sight, hearing, balance, smell, taste, or adaptability to heat and cold is an inevitable part of growing old. Most of the changes, which have been attributed to aging, isn't aging, and is therefore subject to our active review and corrective effort.

Maintaining contact with the world is what life is all about. Insuring that our windows and antennae to that world are clear and in good repair just makes plain good sense. I sincerely hope that the last symphony that I hear will have the same clarity as the symphonies I heard this year, that the last sunset I see will be as luminous as the first, that the bouquet of jasmine is undiminished and the tang of a lemon still sharp, and that my balance remains sturdy and steady until the end. I recognize that having these capacities remain so is largely up to me — and maintaining your senses is largely up to you.

Maintaining Creativity as We Age

Although not one of the five senses, creativity is an important way to keep your sense stimulated and engaged. A creative mind will keep your eyes and ears sharper. The process of creativity provides a focus for all your attention, you see more, hear more, feel more as you expand your experience by creating. However, one of the things you're not supposed to do when you are old is be creative. Much has been written about how persons in their 20s and 30s conceived and delivered most of the worthy creations of history. Ha! This is a widespread misconception that frightens us with the idea that if you haven't done your great work by the time you are 40, then there is no hope for you.

An easy rebuttal to this fallacy is to point out that people simply didn't live much past 40 until recently, and you have a tough time being creative if you're dead. Some people did live to old age and their creativity didn't drop off. Pablo Picasso painted his breakthrough painting *Desmoiselles d'Avignon* at age 26 with a brilliant, creative flourish. *Guernica,* his major humanistic outrage statement, did not occur for 30 more years and reflects a more moral message than the earlier work. Igor Stravinsky wrote the Firebird Suite at 27 years of age, but was producing other mature works into his 80s. Michelangelo similarly showed maturity in his creative development.

I recall a stimulating article in the *New York Times* entitled, "What If Mozart Had Lived?" The writer constructed a logical life history of what Mozart would have amounted to had he lived into his 80s or 90s. As I recall, his career culminated in his appointment as emeritus professor of musicology at Columbia University, having exhaustively explored all sorts of musical avenues in his expanded lifetime. A favorite game is to try to answer the "what if so and so had lived long?" question for lives such as Jesus Christ, Alexander the Great, and John F. Kennedy.

Most of the human experience has been wasted until now because most everyone has died too soon.

Cultivating Creativity

What kinds of strategies can we conceive to maintain the creative spark, and to keep the fires of imagination and innovation as we age? A person is never too young or too old to create. What we create when we're young differs in important aspects from what we create later in life, but both are part of the integrated human experience. A sense in our own competence and capacity to create is essential to creativity at all ages. If we hit a certain calendar year and then sign off on our responsibility to remain creative, I believe our whole life design falls apart and the quality of our later years diminishes.

Here are some tips for staying creative until the day you breathe your last breath:

- ✔ Accept the ongoing responsibility to remain creative by constantly reviewing your skills and needs — reviewing the needs you wish to gratify in filling out your life design and the skills you employ in getting the job done.

- ✔ Believe in your capacity to give something of value that may endure, nurture, teach, and comfort. For example, if you have a flair for gardening, volunteer at your local nursery and teach a class on growing your specialty.

- ✔ Model your effort on those people whom you respect.

- ✔ Test market your ideas for their potential effectiveness.

- ✔ Don't look for guarantees and don't look for what is a sure thing. Look for what *might* become a sure thing. Creativity leaves a rich legacy.

- ✔ Look to the political process. Public policy dictates what kind of world your descendents will live in. Work on it. Writing is a very creative form of expression. If you disagree with a certain political process or policy, write to your congressman.

- ✔ Allow yourself to be surprised.

There is creativity with a capital "C," which applies to those few whose gifts to humanity are widely hailed. But more important is the creativity with a small "c," which stands for all those innumerable acts of bringing new form and reality to the world where previously there was a void or incompleteness. The little "c" creativities range from a garden, to a song, to learning a new language, to making you a more complete person. The process of aging allows time for the completeness of the person, realization of one's potentials, self-actualization.

Chapter 8

Living to Work or Working to Live?

•••

•••

*W*ork helps to define us: "I'm an engineer." "I'm a painter." "I'm a minister." "I'm a dentist." "I'm a teacher." "I'm a cab driver." One of the main things we do in life is work, and in a real sense, work helps to shape us. I can't even imagine what life would be without work — probably dreadful and dangerous, as we would lose much of our purpose.

Because what we do becomes a significant part of who we are, and because work is such a large part of life's design, putting work under the microscope to see what it really is and what effect it has on living longer is crucial.

This chapter explores how our longer lives shape an expanded view of what work is all about. It explores how technology is changing not only the types of work that people do, but the where and for how long. The old definitions of workbench — a 9 a.m. to 5 p.m. workday and a 40-hour workweek — have disappeared to be replaced by extended hours, working at home, flex time, multiple careers, and sabbaticals.

Longer lives mean changing roles as well. Females now find their child-rearing years to be only a small portion of their lives, which gives new opportunity for self-expression and accomplishment. Men and women both find different work agendas. Instead of labor representing lifetimes of calluses and sweat in the factory or home, it increasingly opens multiple broad channels of exploration and discovery about work life.

What's This Thing Called Work?

The main work of all animals involves seeking out and obtaining enough food to stay alive. The threat of starvation brings with it a strong incentive to work. Animals also work to stay warm or stay cool (depending on the climate) and to reproduce (but that's more fun than work).

Anthropologists estimate that present day bushmen and bushwomen spend, on average, 20 to 30 hours per week hunting and gathering food. This modest work week pattern prevailed for hundreds of thousands of generations until the Agricultural Revolution, approximately 10,000 years ago. The shift to farming changed things in many fundamental ways. Populations grew, families were no longer minimally nuclear, and there were more mouths to feed. The Industrial Revolution (about 300 years ago) totally changed the definition of work. The need for food became secondary to the desire for money, power, and more material possessions. Eighty-to 100-hour workweeks became the norm. Soon human existence bore no resemblance to life during the agricultural era. Inventions, such as electric light, spawned longer work hours.

In the late 1800s, labor unions progressively whittled away the long workweeks, against much business resistance. The Great Depression suddenly made work look appealing again, and the wars of the twentieth century also had a way of making people work harder by generating millions of new jobs and bigger paychecks, and as a major byproduct women began sharing the workload. A growing number of people valued money more than free time. The American Dream, including home ownership, emphasized acquiring material goods. Worldwide competition and narrow profit margins drove the workweek up again until it was back at World War I levels of 70 to 80 hours per week — and it continues to grow.

Today's work patterns

People used to work only to satisfy basic needs, but now work supplies much more than that. Theoretically, increased efficiency should yield increased leisure and less work, but the opposite is now the case: We work more and cut back on leisure time. Leisure has decreased 40 percent in 30 years. Wherever choice presents itself, work and income win out. "Shall I spend time with my family, or support it?" is a dilemma felt in millions of homes.

Two recent world events also helped push up the amount of time we spent working. First was the entrance of women to the work force, and second was the graying of the population. Two-thirds of all women are now employed. As the population ages and as people live longer, more and more people are staying in the workforce longer. Even if people retire at 65, they often reenter the workforce in another capacity in a different career.

In today's world, more and more people are choosing to work from their homes. This move away from the office makes lots of sense. It exploits the vast opportunities of the Web, and new technologies continue to evolve that will accelerate this trend. Staying at home enriches family opportunities and provides time for physical exercise, which is often sacrificed by the office routine. Working at home also eliminates one of the main drudges of too many lives, which is commuting (some people's definition of hell). Avoiding the too-long trek to and from work becomes liberating and is good for the environment too.

Working at home encourages men and women to become their own bosses. They can punch their own time clock and write their own paycheck, and most importantly, they can pursue their own dreams rather than someone else's.

The positives of work at home must be balanced by the negatives, boredom and lack of collegial contact. A combination of the two makes a lot of sense.

The positives of work

Having indexed many demerits of work as we now pursue it, listing the positives is important as well. Renowned psychologist Mike Csikszentmihaly's, now at the Claremont Colleges in Southern California, idea of flow (see Chapter 1) places work as the centerpiece of a meaningful life. A Duke University study listed work satisfaction on its short list of factors that predict longevity. Surveys of centenarians constantly reveal the role that work has played in providing significance for their long lives.

Usefulness seems pretty essential to life. Although being useful in this world may be possible without work, getting involved is central to being vital. People often use the phrase "use it or lose it" when they talk about the human body. Without too much of a reach, we can assert that usefulness and vitality are also linked. Being industrious is a key part of a master life strategy.

Work feels good, or at least it should feel good. You should gain some satisfaction from completing an inventory, finishing grading papers, replacing a pipe, contributing a constructive idea, and so forth. Work is — or should be — a challenge. Perhaps the challenge requires new skills, which is another virtue provided by work. Growing in competence feels good.

Often, work satisfaction involves cooperative effort. The pleasure generated by working collectively with others on a common task brings an even greater sense of accomplishment. Being part of a winning team means a shared glory — and the cheers are reinforcing.

Beyond these simple work pleasures comes the recognition that the product of one's labors is making the world better for someone else. The farmer, a druggist, a car salesman, and a bank teller all are gratified when they see their work effort translated into someone else's smile.

Work should feel good, but sometimes it doesn't. Some workdays are dreary, and some work chores are frankly boring. Some workdays are chaotic, and some work tasks are overwhelming. The Greeks had a term "the golden mean," which indicates that for almost everything in life an ideal middle way exists. This certainly applies to the work challenge. Work needs to be busy enough to stimulate and reward, but not too little or too much. Employing the golden mean of work challenge is a constant job for all of us.

Planning ahead helps to avoid the burdens caused by the unexpected stresses of the workday. Making a work schedule can help, as well as clustering certain activities like returning phone or e-mail messages.

How long should you work?

Tote that barge. Lift that bale. Must we dig 'til we drop? For most of history, we have worked until we died. Retirement did not exist. Life expectancy and work expectancy were synonymous. Then Otto von Bismarck, prime minister of Germany in 1880, in a political coup, declared that Germans over the age of 65 were entitled to a pension. Of course, this was easy for him to say because it ensured his political power by simply retiring his opponents, most of whom were over 65. Bismarck declared a new human right — the right to stop working on a certain arbitrary birthday. The idea was such a stroke of political genius that I wonder why no one had thought of it before!

Retirement became such a seductive idea that the rest of the industrialized world clamored to jump on the bandwagon. When people in the United States inaugurated their Social Security system, 40 other workers supported the one person collecting a Social Security check. Today, three workers support each recipient, and soon the ratio will be one to one. Given these trends, it is important for you to plan now for your own retirement — physically, emotionally, and financially.

Figuring out how long you should work means creating a time/interest/obligation/financial budget for the rest of your life. Sure, money matters, but other dimensions of your future life are just as, or maybe more, important. Someone suggested that one way of approaching the task of future time and effort allocation is to write your own obituary. How would you like it to read? Do you want it to reveal that you are the richest guy or gal in the cemetery? Certainly not. But you would want it to include major mention of your family involvement. You would likely record your career efforts and the good effects that they had in your community. But beyond work and family you would like to brag about who else you were or are.

You taught Sunday school. You were a birdwatcher. You volunteered in the emergency room. You were active in your civic organization. You contributed to charity. You loved your dog. You were healthy until you died.

These "what else" parts of your life work budget should guide your decisions. Life is work, but it is more than work. Many people discover parts of themselves that they haven't had a chance to develop after their work demands cease. They become "more me."

Paying Your Way in Life

Life is not free. Despite what the songs may tell you, the best things in life are the things you work for. Mandatory retirement and enforced inactivity present dangers. Did you know that in 1948, 50 percent of potential workers over 65 stayed on the job, while only 16 percent did in 1987? Fewer and fewer of us are found doing the same work tasks we did 20 or 30 or 50 years before. The paychecks are certain to bear different signatures, but for most of us the notion of continuing involvement with life, as signified by a productive, if different, life course is a potent and sustaining force. Idleness doesn't make sense — or cents.

Pretend that you are going to live to be 100. When I put this projection to several financial planners, they simply shriek and throw up their hands at the prospect. But what if this assumption is correct? Can you currently afford to live to be 100? If not, then how are you going to do so?

 I recoil at the idea of becoming a "DUMPY" — a word coined to denote a destitute, unemployed, mature, person. I give many lectures to senior organizations, hospitals, insurance companies, retirement communities, and corporations and beat my chest about the future glories that growing old can hold for us. Often, I get a rousingly enthusiastic response. The biggest stumbling block, however, is when my listeners realize that "I can't afford to live to be 100." You can afford to live that long — but you need to plan now. You can't afford to think you will depend on Social Security.

Plan on working longer

First, we need to work longer. Several friends and I calculated on a paper napkin that to afford to be 100, we will need to work until we are 80.

Most experts agree that productive employment and family relationships are the two things that older persons hold most valuable in their treasure bank. If this is so, we should sustain both jobs and family as late into life as possible. We cherish the opportunity to remain valuable and necessary. We accomplish this by continuing to work and staying engaged in the mainstream of life. Work guarantees involvement and provides the most congenial setting for "flow" (see Chapter 1).

Asserting that a good (if unusual) survival strategy is to reset your retirement calendar to age 80 does not imply that you need to continue flipping burgers or making widgets until you are four-score years old. Circling age 80 on your future calendar simply gives you the chance to develop meaningful opportunities for a productive enterprise now. It gives you added responsibility for yourself today — and additional opportunities for the future.

Start saving now

So the first step in assuring financial solvency in your trip to 100 is to continue to work until you are 80. That solves most of the problems right away. But beyond this, you should save — and start as soon as you possibly can.

My best advice?

- ✔ Burn your credit card when you are 50 and start paying cash.
- ✔ Be aggressive in your investment strategy.
- ✔ Investigate reverse mortgages and charitable remainder trusts and annuities, as they can allow you extraordinary late-life latitude.
- ✔ Check in with a financial planner to see how you can save for your future and still enjoy your life today. Many older people certainly do not want to become a financial burden to their children and other family members — some to the point of neglecting their own needs while they are still relatively young and active. But with the proper combination of planning, advice, and investments, enjoying your golden years and still providing a comfortable nest egg for when you might need it most is possible.

For more specific information on planning for your retirement, check out *Personal Finance For Dummies* or *Retirement Planning For Dummies* (both published by Hungry Minds, Inc.).

As a geriatrician, I have presided over the deaths of several thousand older persons. Almost without exception, the death moment, which should be of exquisite sensitivity for all, is instead a "what do we do now?" scene. This includes financial matters. Please, write the script for your last act in advance, and make sure the involved persons have rehearsed for their roles. Pretending that any of us can remain autonomous until the very end is foolish. Hopefully, the last song will be brief, but however long it is, the last song should be a chorus and not a solo.

Avoiding Four Common Retirement Traps

Seeing that the last act of life is well written and well played calls for a new competency, because the plot is all-new. People have never lived this long before. People have never had a chance to retire before. No wild animal has a retirement plan or rest home assigned. How we manage this last act often determines the way other people will remember us, so doing it well is important.

If you assume that work expectancy is planned as 80 years for a life expectancy of 100 years, that still leaves 20 years for retirement. Where do you turn for advice on how to spend those last 20 years? You can begin by avoiding the following mistakes that many others have made before you.

1. **I've got lots of time left. When my time comes, I'll figure out what I'll be doing when I walk away from the workbench.**

   Wrong. If you arrive on the first day of the rest of your life with no clue as to what the rest of your life may be, that day and all those that follow it will be pitiful shells of what they should be. Retirement, like anything that is really important, needs a lot of planning. The sooner you start your planning, the better. Having a firm handle on the timing is crucial. Beyond that, a careful inventory of your interests and skills will open up many new doors. Look around at what others are doing. Read the papers. Do research on the Internet. Start planning what to do with the rest of your life before you pull out of the office parking lot for your last commute home.

2. **Of course I'll have enough money to retire. I'll get around to finances next year.**

   Wrong, wrong, wrong. Retirement places new parameters on a budget. Some expenses will go down, while others will go up. Retirement financial planning is a whole new world. You will certainly not lack for eager people waiting to tell you how to finance the rest of your life, but usually such persons are really looking for ways to finance the rest of their lives. Only you can place priorities and make those very personal allotments of cash and energy. Your children and families should be involved in creating the overall strategy, because they should be partners in your last years, as you were in their first years.

3. **The doctors will take care of my health.**

   Wrong. You are your own best doctor. We physicians are here for the moment when you need us, but you are the one around for the long haul. Health is largely determined by your behavior, and you — not your physician — control your health decisions. Physicians cannot act as your health proxy. Your physician needs explicit instructions about your wishes for your last moments and how you choose to spend them. Until that final shepherding comes about, however, you control your present and future health.

4. **I'll probably move to the south when I retire.**

   Wrong. Climate is one of the least important determinants of where you should retire. Yes, you should plan some travel to warm up in the sun periodically, but your last nest should probably be close to where your present one is, and probably the same one. Where you have lived your life is where you have spent most of your energies. Where you live is likely most accommodating to what you really need and want from life, and where your major competencies reside.

If you do move with retirement, I recommend that you move closer to your children — whether or not they live in a warm climate. If your children have been a major part of your past life, they should be a major part of your future life. A great priority in retirement is grandparenting and great-grandparenting. Who else better deserves the best products of your life experiences than your flesh and blood? Don't think warm; think home and family.

Staying Active and Challenged upon Retirement

We now know that the old paradigm of life is worn out. Spending early life in school, midlife at work and with the family, and late life in the rocking chair just doesn't work anymore. This sequence is way out of synch with both the future and the present. The first crucial element that figures in your new life structure is how long you are going to live — and that's a lot longer than you had thought. Our present allocation of lifetime for education and work time is predicated on models created one hundred or more years ago when people died young. Going to school until you are 18 or 22 is okay if you are going to be dead by 45. Work time and planning for retirement at 65 or 60 is okay if you are embalmed by 65, but what if you are going to live to be 100 and you have read your last book 80 years ago, or cashed your last paycheck 35 years ago? Does that make any sense at all?

The new 100-year lifetime demands a reorganization of life segments. Instead of a linear sequence of education, work, and leisure, these three segments need to be integrated over all ten decades. Each decade from one to ten should include the same three basic elements: training, action, and contemplation. Each segment should continuously nourish the other. Instead of monolithic long blocks of time, we will derive a dynamic interactive process, a set of sabbatical experiences drawing from other capacities and then moving on. Instead of long periods of equilibrium, we will initiate punctuations of change in which new experience is encouraged to interact with new training and new reflections so that life can grow at a continual rate until its terminus. Instead of boredom or stress, we will live in a lifetime of flow opportunity in which new skills and new challenges constantly interplay.

One of my favorite observations says, "If who you are is what you do, when you don't you aren't." This aphorism connects doing to being. This tie is powerful. What the saying doesn't assert, however, is what does "doing" mean? Does it mean continued dreary years in boring pursuits, or, more hopefully, can "doing" convey a sense of lifelong involvement in things that really matter. Next, you might ask, "What does 'matter' mean?" Every living person (or who has ever or will ever live) probably has a different answer to that question. Some individual answers to what matters have higher values than do others. Find what matters to you, whether it be reading a new novel every month or volunteering at your local hospital once a week, and take the time to do it!

Later life means not only more years, but more time in each day — more "free" time. This "free time" can matter, depending on how you spend it. Older persons have developed an extensive repertoire of competence. Programs such as the Retired Senior Volunteer Program (RSVP), seek to keep the competence of retired people in harness. The options for retired people are many and varied: the Peace Corps, environmental protections, the education enterprise, political participation such as city council or committees, health aids, and so forth.

Lives, like muscles, are meant to be used. Some late-life activities may involve payment, many others don't. In either case, payment is not the principal issue; doing something and staying engaged is.

Further, making your late-life years matter may involve personal as well as worldly tasks. Learning to play a musical instrument, or a new language, or new skills (computer use immediately comes to mind), or improving your health all count toward extending your "mattering" quotient.

Through these goals, life derives a richer texture. Rather than retirement representing a constriction of life, it should become an expansion. Someone observed that the really important question is not "What are you retiring from?" but "What are you retiring to?" Retirement should be like graduation — an opening up of unexplored talents, interests, and opportunities. A whole new world waits for you out there.

This new exploration may exploit capacities that you have already worked to develop. You may develop a consulting service to share your competence. You may join organizations such as the Experience Corps or RSVP, which exists to take advantage of your talents. You may want to start a spin-off business. Nothing flashy, but simply the chance to work out a hidden idea that you haven't had the time to explore.

Perhaps your retirement urges you to seek out altogether new areas. Music, travel, language, public service, and history are all rich domains that exist for your exploration. The World Wide Web gives instant access to all sorts of enticing prospects. And the cost is relatively cheap too.

Chapter 9

Sex Matters

● ●

In This Chapter

▶ Seeing sex in old and new ways

▶ Keeping sex alive for life

● ●

*1*f you're going to live a long time, it makes good sense to get a handle on the basic drives that make life happen. Eating, breathing, and moving come to mind immediately. And sex?

High up on the list of reasons that people use to claim they don't want to live to be 100 is diminished sex life. They imagine themselves as frail shells of their former selves who would not only be physically incapable of a sex life, but probably not interested, either.

Yes, your sex life will change, but thank goodness! It certainly changed between adolescence and age 40, didn't it? The key is to enjoy what you can do at every age. And that's exactly what this chapter is all about — ways to keep the romance in your relationship alive and methods for handling some of the directions that your sex life might evolve toward as you age. For more detailed information on these topics, check out *Sex For Dummies* or *Rekindling Romance For Dummies* (both published by Hungry Minds, Inc.).

 Old people can. Old people do. In fact, several scientific reports indicate that if you really are planning to be 100, having a good sex life is a good place to start.

In this chapter, I build the premise that life-long sexual activity is not only possible but also desirable. I review the recent science behind this perspective and document the positive aspects of late-life sexuality. In so doing, I don't neglect or obscure the large amount of negative imagery associated with sex and aging, but I do hope to place it in context and to provide action steps you can take to prevent the sad and usually inaccurate predictions. The widespread myth exists that sex belongs exclusively to the younger generations. This idea has been thoroughly and thankfully demolished by numerous surveys. Not only do old people maintain a robust and lively interest in sex, but, more importantly, they follow their urges.

Exposing the Lie

In the past, when questions would arise from patients and listeners in lecture audiences about sexual matters, I would stumble badly. In an effort to get on the stick and repair this ignorance, I read and studied everything I could, but still felt inadequate. So, I decided to put on a public forum on the topic. Several colleagues and I advertised a three-evening series about sex and aging to be held at our local senior center.

As the first evening approached I wondered "What if no one shows up?" I needn't have worried because the place was packed, and, interestingly, most of the audience was male. This contrasts most lectures on aging topics where the attendees are largely female. The average age of our audience of nearly 200 was 68, and they were acutely attentive throughout. The majority of the attendees were married or had a sexual partner. Our expert panel went over topics ranging from anatomy and function to disease and drugs — everything was on display. Questions and concerns bubbled up. At the end of the series, we handed out a questionnaire about attitudes and performance. Completing the questionnaire was voluntary and anonymous, but most everyone sent it back. The responses revealed two major findings. First, the group was very interested in sex and was busily pursuing this interest. Second, the group's sexual interest and performance were both burdened by numerous problems — some of which were predictable and others of which were totally unexpected in nature.

First the good news

Ninety-two percent of our lecture group reported that ideally they would wish to have sex once per week. This figure was similar for men and women, and for those less and more than 70 years of age. Interestingly, this preferred frequency conformed to that of the attendees' reported practices 10 years earlier, but was notably less than currently practiced. In other words, both the men and women wished for more frequent sexual encounters than they were experiencing.

The male respondents placed a higher value upon intercourse as their preferred form of sexual activity, whereas the females rated "loving and caring" most highly. This observation is reminiscent of an aging/sex study at Duke University several years ago in which male respondents seemed to place more emphasis on the quantity of their sexual encounters, while the females indicated a more persistent interest in the quality of the encounters.

Despite the generally lusty attitude and activities of our evening group, we did note a clear fall in frequency of sexual expression with age. Sixty percent of the group indicated a decrease in sexual performances in the last 10 years, 32 percent indicated no change, and 8 percent indicated an increase. These statistics are similar from those of a larger study conducted 15 years ago. In this report performed by the public interest group Consumers' Union, 73, 63, and 50 percent of women in their fifties, sixties, and seventies, respectively, reported having intercourse at least once per week. Correspondingly, the percentages were 90, 73, and 58 for the same decades in men. Further, 50 percent of the men over 80 in this group recorded sexual activity at least once per week.

The critic will ask, "How do you know these figures are not all exaggerations?" The answer is, "You can't know for sure, but checks within the questionnaires reflect an internal consistency, and thereby provide confidence in the meaning of the results." What is more certain about the figures, however, is that they are very likely to change as societal attitudes change. An 80-year-old of today is a very different person, sexually and in other ways, than the 80-year-old of 50 years from now. I can only predict that the sexual numbers cited in the previous paragraph will increase.

Several experts have commented on the relative stability of sexuality over the life span, which means that if you and your mate had a vigorous approach to sex in your 20s, you'll likely carry on that trend until late in life. The old saying of "use it or lose it" is affirmed again. This constancy does not, however, account for the substantial numbers of older men and women who report that their sexual profiles in late life are better than they have been. Psychiatrist Eric Pfeiffer wrote that 20 percent of older men feel their sexual lives are better than they were at younger ages.

Sexuality sits wonderfully at the intersection of the biological, psychological, and sociological domains of life. All three are active participants in a wholesome sexual life. Although it is unlikely that biologic change with age would likely confer any advantage to older persons (other than the possible relief from anxiety about possible pregnancy that accompanies a menopause), it is very possible that a great variety of psychological and social adjustments occur with aging that could predictably enhance sexuality.

From a strictly biologic and reproductive point of view, sex is best left to the young. This conception is based on the indisputable fact that age provokes gene change that has major implications for family planning. Whereas only 1 in 526 20-year-old women show chromosomal defects in their ovaries, this frequency rises to 1 in 7 for 49-year-old women. Determination of male sperm chromosomal pattern is less sternly age affected.

These are interesting and important facts, but they should not obscure the fact that, for humans, reproduction is only a very secondary component of sexual activity. For most of us, sex represents the ultimate in social bonding. It generates long-term commitments, respect, and devotion. It encourages mutual spiritual growth. All of the psychosocial roles that sex plays in us humans do not diminish, in fact should enlarge, as the decades pass.

The flush and rush of early chemical infatuation is on most dramatic display in young lovers, but old lovers can twinkle too. On the other hand, the fine polish that only late-life companionship offers is a deeper and more enduring gift.

So, sure, age matters with sexuality. Along with the well-documented decrements of sexual performance, however, come opportunities for sustaining a long and caring relationship into the tenth decade and beyond.

Now, the bad news

The first "sex practice in aging" survey I did, mentioned earlier in the chapter, showed clearly that our older subjects both thought about and acted upon sex more than was expected. The second strong finding was that problems do exist. Both men and women have problems. Eighty-five percent of the men under 70 (79 percent of those over 70) and 63 percent of the women under 70 (44 percent of the women over 70) reported that they were either somewhat or very troubled by some aspects of their sex lives. What were the problems? For men, the difficulty expressed was nearly exclusively confined to impotency. For the women, the problems had more to do with social rather than biologic issues.

To explore in more depth the troubled male, I initiated another large survey, this time exclusively with men. Through lectures and a number of retired men's luncheon clubs a sample of 1,202 men was obtained. The average age of the respondents was 73.8, with 18 percent over the age of 80. A 63-item questionnaire asked assorted questions dealing with present and past sexual attitudes and practices.

Once again, a falloff in average sexual activity was noted. The 55 to 59 year age group reported a median value of 3.6 times per month for sexual intercourse, while the 85 to 94 year age group reported only 1.3 times per month. Great variance existed within these groups. Five percent of the 228 men over 80 years of age reported having intercourse two or more times per week, and an additional 12 percent had intercourse at least once per week. There was, therefore, a subset of the older men to whom the declines did not seem to apply.

We asked why. Three answers emerged. First, these lusty 80-year-olds had good physical health, second they took few if any medicines, and third they had a willing and loving partner. We termed this group our "exemplars." They represented the reality that for a substantial number of older men impotency and diminished sex lives are not in fact inevitable.

I published these results in the May 1999 issue of the *Journal of Gerontology*. The conclusion stated, "These findings negate a portion of the starkly negative imagery of sexual expression in aging males." It is therefore heartening to be able to state boldly that there is hope, that impotence is not the sure fate of us guys as we age.

The fact remains however that the great majority of older men suffer from some degree of impotence.

Handling Sexual Difficulties

The handful of scientific projects designed to look into the topic of sex and aging are in agreement on several findings. First, older people are more sexually active than is generally appreciated. In one report, college students estimated that their parents made love three times per month. The actual frequency was seven times. One-quarter of the students guessed that their parents never made love.

Second, consistency of lifestyle predicts late-life sexuality. If sex is an important component of earlier life quality, it is more likely to be sustained into late life. Twenty percent of older men feel that their sex lives are better than earlier in life. Women too report lessened tensions, inhibitions, and better communication about sex in their upper decades.

Third, problems do exist. Identifying that you may have a problem is key to ensuring a long and healthy sex life. For men the principal difficulties involve impotence. For women it involves lack of opportunity. Illness, death, and medication use make men less able and available consorts for women.

Male sexuality and aging

As we men age, we age in many ways. Among the most important is our sexuality. Both in terms of desire (libido) and performance, we simply aren't the same person as 10 or 50 years ago. Some aspects, such as having more leisure time and lowered performance pressures, are conducive to improved sexuality. Other features, biologic ones, are negative. The most common of these is impotence.

Millions of older men acknowledge various degrees of difficulty in achieving or maintaining an erection. Only recently have scientists begun to understand the biology of having an erection. Doctors have always known that an erection results when the penis fills with blood, but the specific mechanism was totally unknown. Now we know.

The little molecule that dilates blood vessels wherever they are in the body is nitric oxide. It is the active ingredient in nitroglycerine, which is a widely used little pill for the treatment of heart pain (angina). When the heart arteries are constricted, the heart becomes starved for blood and a crushing chest pain results. Put a nitro pill under the tongue and "ah, relief" as the nitric oxide relaxes the arteries and allows the blood to flow again. Frequently headaches accompany the use of the pill because it is not smart enough only to dilate the heart arteries and dilates the ones in the head too. Because scientists know how nitric oxide works on arteries all over the body, concluding that nitric oxide initiates an erection was not much of a leap of logic.

Initial efforts to apply a salve or cream of nitric oxide to the penis to cause an erection failed because the cream's time of action was too short. Consequently, compounds that generate nitric oxide when ingested (first alprostadil and, more recently, Viagra) entered the market. Viagra's introduction represented the single most explosive new drug in history. (I wish I had bought stock.) The Pfizer Company discovered Viagra's effect as an accident. The drug was initially promoted as a blood pressure lowering medication, but it didn't work very well. As a result, Pfizer decided to recall all the samples that had been distributed as part of the mass testing of any new drug. They were surprised when the men refused to send back the samples. Hence, Pfizer had a big winner, unexpectedly. Viagra has been a very successful drug for men with erectile dysfunction (to use Bob Dole's term). Rarely, there have been fatalities associated with its use, although some have occurred particularly with men who are taking nitroglycerine simultaneously (not a good idea). Always seek advice from your physician prior to taking any medication — never "try" other's medications.

Impotence occurs because collagen deposits in the vascular channels of the penis and clogs them up. The answer to this problem is to get rid of the collagen by having an erection. Erections are good for erections. The principle of "use it or lose it" is again affirmed. There probably should be a RDA (recommended daily allotment) of erections for maintaining good erectile competence.

For men the ability to have an erection is much more than a biologic event. It is identifying. It is a life competence. It is an essential marker of the intactness of our ego. In addition to the previously mentioned new knowledge about the mechanical details that produce an erection, there has been extensive sober reflection on *all* the factors that bear on this capacity, including:

- ✔ **Boredom.** Freshness, variety, and excitement are part of the environment for good sexuality. Make an effort to keep sex adventuresome and new.

- ✔ **Preoccupation with money or career.** I can testify that anxiety over a job dispute or an IRS review is a stern disincentive to a good sex life. You need to check these concerns at the bedroom door.

- ✔ **Fatigue.** Exhaustion from heavy physical or mental labor is not a good setting for sexual adequacy. An erection, after all, requires a concentration of blood in the penis. If it is all puddled up in tired tissues, it is unavailable for erection purposes. Sex works best when not wiped out.

✔ **Stress.** Our days seem fuller and fuller, and faster and faster. Good erections take time and space. Stress releases endorphins that mess with the sex hormones.Crowding our lives with all sorts of frenzy is a poor idea of a good sex life.

✔ **Alcohol.** Booze and erections don't mix. Even Shakespeare knew that, "Alcohol provokes the desire, but dulls the performance." Alcohol is a depressant. It dulls perception and performance. Millions of promising sexual encounters have faltered because alcohol deflated the penis.

✔ **Depression.** A glum outlook does not serve having adequate erections. Sexual excitement simply is inconsistent with a dim world view. A fit person is not a depressed person, and vice versa.

✔ **Unwilling partner.** Loving receptivity is the logical co-partner to potency. It is the bilateral bonding contract that intercourse should represent. Failure of either partner to show their commitment is a no-go.

✔ **Fear of failure.** Every man has had the exasperating experience of erectile failure just when it shouldn't have occured. These misadventures are haunting, and regardless of their cause, remain as worries — "Could it happen again?" This phobia feeds on itself and may require therapeutic intervention if it persists.

✔ **Health problems.** The list is long of medical conditions that can adversely affect erectile competence. The penis is a vascular organ, so anything that produces poor blood flow can adversely affect erection. Diabetes is at the head of the list, but the list of illnesses affecting erections could fill a page. A urologist is the medical specialist most qualified to investigate impotence.

✔ **Medication use.** Some of the most gratifying experiences I have had as a physician have involved the discovery that some particular medication was messing with my haunted patient's sexual competence. Simply reducing the dose, or switching to an alternative medication is always met by a broad grin of appreciation. Most primary care physicians are aware of the adverse sexual side effects that many medicines may cause. Don't be embarrassed to ask.

✔ **Prostate problems.** Although the prostate gland is not directly involved with producing an erection, its anatomic proximity causes it to become a consideration when listing factors relating to male sexual function. This lime-sized gland lies deep in our pelvis, at the outlet of the bladder where the urethra emerges. Its function is to make the fluid in which the sperm are suspended. It does not make testosterone; that important compound is made by the testicles. The size of the prostate is sensitive to the action of testosterone, however.

The prostate presents two problems to the older male. The first goes by the name of benign prostatic hypertrophy (BPH for short). This non-malignant enlargement causes a gradual swelling of the prostate so that it takes up too much of the volume of the urinary bladder or it may actually shut off the urethral urine flow. The common symptoms have to do with urinating — excessive, difficult, or nocturnal. Surgery is the current principal treatment of this non-life threatening but distressing condition. The other prostate worry is cancer. Magazine covers, TV specials, and ad campaigns all detail what seems to be an alarming increase in incidence of this condition. Some of the increased incidence, however, is due to the availability of the simple blood test, prostate specific antigen (PSA), which is very helpful in detection. This test should be on the required list of annual physical exams for men in the 65 to 80 year age group. Multiple treatment options are available, and require having a good, caring physician.

Female sexuality and aging

And what about women? The truth is, the scientific community knows even less about women than men. While the male problem is largely mechanical, the female issues are much more complex with biologic, psychologic, and social factors all interplaying. Betty Friedan's book *Fountain of Age* includes an excellent chapter on intimacy issues of older women, which describes with much sensitivity the lack of conceptual framework from which advisories can be derived. If desire is low (libido), testosterone is of proven value for women as it is for men. Several preparations, including skin patch and a cream, can raise the sexual interest of older women. Hormone replacement with estrogen and progesterone is now widely advised for older women for a variety of reasons, not the least of which is the facilitating of good health of the female sexual tissues. Lack of estrogen commonly promotes atrophic vaginitis, which is often a stern disincentive for sexual activity.

The main event in the older woman's sexual life is her menopause. Once again, the cessation of menstrual periods has much more than biologic significance. It signals the end of reproductive capacity, which for many women is central to their life role. For many women this loss is profound, while for others it is a relief or liberation.

The loss of monthly production of estrogen has real biologic meaning. It is no accident that until menopause, women (unless they are smokers) are virtually immune to heart attacks. The menopause signals the end of their immunity. Estrogens have been implicated too in the protective effects against osteoporosis. Alzheimer's disease is also nominated as a condition that may be ameliorated by hormone replacement therapy.

What, to me, was a very strong story supporting these estrogens in post-menopausal women for the three indications mentioned previously has been modified by several large epidemiologic surveys that were less than enthusiastic in their results. Therefore, in my opinion, we are in a "wait for more evidence" mode before endorsing widespread use of estrogens after the menopause.

The value of estrogen taken either orally or applied locally for thinned and sensitive genital tissues is beyond dispute. Analysis of female adequacy for satisfactory late-life sexual activity is far less studied or revealing than for the man. Clearly, tender tissues is easily remedied. Less easily solved, however, are the issues of lack of interest and lack of opportunity. "I don't really care about sex" is obviously not an attitude that leads to a promising sex life. When I hear this lament, I do not blithely and respectfully defer to it. To me, sexuality is a huge quality of life issue for women as well as for men, and anyone who shuts this out, with or without good reason, is a sorrow. When one of my patients says to me, "I don't feel like exercising," I don't accept that verdict, I try to change it. So, too, if disinterest in sex appears in a female patient, I try my clumsy best to address it. If I fail, however, I am quick to advise consultation with a sex therapist.

I acknowledge that this aggressive approach to the younger-older lady has some rationale, but I am troubled by the appropriateness of my urging to a 90-year-old who may have been widowed for 15 years. Accepting the reality of this situation, I nonetheless cling to my ideal that life is to be lived fully and robustly until its last ember dies, hopefully after your 100th birthday. And this fully robust life connotes some form of sexuality and intimacy, even when the odds are stacked against it.

The other negative older female sexuality issue is simply numerical. There aren't enough of us older guys to go around. The simple answer to this quandary is for the men to live longer so that the ratio is more equal. Yet, lacking a slick answer to this suggestion, we are stuck with a statistical imbalance. Fortunately, women, lacking men, appear to turn to other older women in the same predicament in which they find themselves for companionship and understanding. Women bond with other women much more comfortably than men bond with men. It bothers me a lot that when a wife dies, the husband's mortality is at great risk. On the other hand, when a husband dies, the widow seems not to be threatened by his absence.

I am struck by the term "social convoy." This term reflects the circle of intimate contacts most of us surround ourselves with as life winds its way. Our individual social convoy is a major survival tool. Those who lack it simply don't live as long. Women are notably more adept at constituting and maintaining their social convoy.

The majority of age/sexuality features listed under male issues in the previous section (boredom, depression, stress, fatigue, alcohol, health and medicine, and spousal incompatibility) also conspire to diminish the quality of an older woman's responsiveness. All of these issues apply to women, and they matter a great deal.

A sad but true observation is in order. We physicians are abominably bad in dealing with sexual issues with our older patients. We are embarrassed, ignorant, and threatened. We, as a profession, have a great deal of maturing to do to deal effectively with this important issue.

Keeping the Flame Alive

Instead of late-life sexuality representing a dying ember, soon to extinguish, it should be thought of as a lingering warmth that requires tending to ensure continued flame and sparks. This cannot happen casually. It takes planning and mutual commitment.

All those complications which crowd the quiet romantic moments — congested housing, medication use, arthritis, grandchildren — have solutions. Don't forget that earlier in this chapter (under "Now the bad news"), I wrote about the "sexual exemplars" whom we identified in our research study. Although our study group was exclusively older males, I am confident that the same qualifying attributes apply to older women as well.

In order to be a sexual exemplar as you age, first you need good health. This is largely under your personal control with your physician's assistance. Careful attention to medication use is critical. Important too is creating the time and space for intimacy. Here are some tips for connecting with your significant other:

- Enjoying a romantic dinner

- Going on a weekend getaway

- Finding activities you both enjoy and doing them together

- Renewing wedding vows

- Making a special celebration for anniversaries, birthdays, and so on

- Checking out *Sex For Dummies* and *Rekindling Romance For Dummies,* both by Dr. Ruth Westheimer (Hungry Minds, Inc.)

Every older person can summon up from deeply stored memories images of a full moon over the water, or the last slow dance at the prom, or smooching in the back seat at a drive-in movie, or the smell of perfumed hair, or a corsage, or self-conscious love notes — the list goes on and on. But the point is: Are these memories necessarily confined to the awkward and often anxious teenage years, or can romance linger into the present? Love need not go stale with time, but, like a successful garden, it needs plenty of attention. If recalling those infatuated moments still can give goose bumps of pleasure, why not rekindle these embers? No one is ever too old to deny the delight of candlelight dinners, or an unexpected present, or a massage, or a sweet love song. Wedding anniversaries provide perfect opportunities for rededication and rediscovery of the sweet moments. Being healthy and happy together is the "right stuff." Romance makes the rest of the world glow brighter. It boosts common energies and enhances longevity.

Sex Can Extend Your Life

Sex is a large part of quality of life at any age, young and old. Evidence even suggests that sex might extend your life. In 1997 an article appeared in the British Medical Journal entitled "Sex and Death, Are They Related?" It concerned a survey of 1,222 men aged 45 to 59 from Caerphilly, South Wales. After 10 years, 150 of the men had died. The sexually active group had half the mortality of the sexually inactive group.

As I hope for my eyes, ears, heart, legs to be fully functional until my terminal decline, so too do I hope that my sexual flames still burns brightly until the end. Aging brings advantages to sexuality and sexuality gives polish to the image of aging. It maintains bonding. It is virtual communication. It is affirming. It is smarter, less urgent, and more honest. Sustaining sexuality, as sustaining physical exercise, should be a common life goal. The more informed we become about aspects of our basic nature, the more capable we will become of finishing life as we started — with bright eyes and a tender heart.

Females outlive males

One of the persistent and troubling aspects of late-life sexuality is the numerical disparity of older women and men. This is due to the well-documented spread in life expectancies between the two sexes.

Why do women outlive men? My mother was a widow for 22 years after my father died. Although the length of her widowhood exceeded the usual duration of seven or eight years, such a prolonged loneliness is not rare. What is the explanation for women's longevity advantage? There is no clear answer to this simple question, but there are many conjectures. It seems that Mother Nature places a higher value on the lives of her female descendents than on those of her sons. This advantage is widely seen throughout all creatures.

I read an interesting speculation that noted that in those species in which the male is an active partner in child rearing, the gender/life span disparity is less than in those more common circumstances in which the male fulfills his biologic role by sperm donation, and is never heard from again. Nurturance and longevity sound like they should go together.

Others speculate that the reason men die too soon is our bad health habits. Until recently, smoking was mostly a male habit. Unfortunately, however, its embrace by women has diminished their immunity to smoking-induced illnesses — and the death certificates give grim evidence of this fact.

My own best guess as to why women outlive us guys has to do with their coping abilities. Women bend, men break. Women are supple, men are rigid. Women tend to their health better than men do. They use their doctors and healthcare system better than men do.

Interestingly, speculation exists that as men age they become more feminine in perspective and in biology. As the male testosterone levels fall with age, men become less irascible, less confrontational, and nicer (or so the theory goes). It would certainly make a neater and more balanced world if men's longevity equaled women's.

Sex as exercise

Implicit in any discussion of late-life sexuality is a concern that the exertion encountered during sex may be the tipping point to an otherwise frail person. What would people think if grandpa died while. . . ?! To give you a reference point, intercourse is roughly equivalent in terms of exercise intensity to climbing a flight of stairs. The risk of heart attacks in a low-risk person is about 1 per 1 million hours. Sexual activity doubles this to 2 per 1 million hours.

This is an extremely small risk. Further, you can totally offset the risk by being physically fit — another credential to add to the benefit list of physical exercise. I surveyed sexual habits of the members of the physically active Fifty Plus Fitness Association. This group is known for having a disability and mortality rate that is only 30 percent of the national average. The male and female members of our extremely physically active group reported above average sexual interest and activity. Which causes which? Do the members live longer because they are sexually active, or does their physical activity confer late-life sexual competency?

Looking into the mirror

This whole chapter and the entire topic of late-life sexuality are extremely important to me personally. As a healthy 70-year-old male, I thank my stars that I live in the era of sexual illumination. No longer are these topics hidden from public and even private review. Sex is labeled, properly, as a central quality of life issue for people of all ages. It pervades every corner of our lives. It can anguish, but it can exalt. I prefer the latter, and the more we know the less the anguish will be.

Our first 1996 sex and aging study reporting the results of a small seminar asked first about the amount of sexuality older people experience, second how we feel about it, and third and most importantly can anything be done to improve it? The results of our and other information leads to three responses. First, older people maintain a largely unrecognized vigorous interest in and pursuit of sexual pleasures until late in life. Second, those who fail, for many reasons, feel their sexual experience to be less than they would wish for and are upset by it. Third, their unhappiness is approachable, and, in many ways, improvable.

Being healthy, sexually, and in all other ways is under your personal control. Responding to this reality makes sense.

Chapter 10

Building Your Last Nest

In This Chapter

▶ Staying near your support convoy

▶ Making end-of-life decisions rationally

▶ Staying involved 'til the end

*W*hen it comes to living a long, full life, the first question most people ask is, "How?" (Well, sometimes the question is, "Why?" but earlier chapters of this book answer the skeptics.) One question many neglect to ask is just as important: "Where?" Where you decide to live out the last decades of your life constitutes a huge part of how happy you will be. People who are unhappy with where they are living have a shorter life span — although even a short life span may seem an eternity if you don't like your last nest. This chapter explores the factors that impact your decision about where you will live in your future. I like to call it your "omega home."

Grappling with the New Mobility

Where to live as we age is a new question. During most of history, when people got older, they simply stayed where they always had been — with their families. Having kids was the social security system, and is still the system in the developing world. Even in developed nations such as Japan, one-third of older people live in three-generation households. In the United States, however, only one percent of older people still do. In Japan, two-thirds of older people live with their children, in Britain, France, and the U.S. only one-sixth do. The single-person households in the United States have skyrocketed, from 5 percent in 1900 to 13 percent in 1960 and 25 percent today. Many of these households are older people. Housing questions during the end decades of life are new — and unique to the western world.

The modern world has become so mobile that it has disrupted the old patterns. According to *USA Today,* people move every seven or eight years. I have two friends who have no home at all, pausing in a central hotel room periodically to restock. Nomads have always existed, but that lifestyle required that the older generations kept pace with the movers so that they weren't left behind. A recent Del Webb national survey indicated that 43 percent of baby boomers believed that they would move sometime in their future, and of those, 14 percent thought that they would move out of state. The boomers are in contrast with only 4 percent of the current retired population who see an out-of-state move and only 14 percent who foresee any move at all.

The parent-child bond into middle age and later

With whom you spend your last years is no longer as clear as it once was. Historically, you would spend those years with your children and grandchildren. Today, however, mobility has created a new sense of independence, but has also made our roots less deep and lessened the focus on long-lasting commitments. The relationship of middle-aged people with their parents and their own children has spawned the term "the sandwich generation." People feel caught between the old patterns of family interdependency and the fresh concept of individual freedom. For some, the sense of responsibility for one's parents suffers under this conflict.

When considering any move away from family, know that there will likely be major hurts that result. Never undertake a move without calculating in all the costs, particularly the emotional ones.

As in all relationships, the parent-child relationship swings back and forth. In the beginning, the children take. In the end, the parents must take. Pete Peterson's book *Gray Dawn* gives census data indicating that 25- to 34-year-olds receive 20 times as much financial support from their parents as they give. Even 35- to 44-year-olds receive five times more support than they give. Even into middle age, parents are actively involved in their children's well-being.

And what about 20, 30, and 40 years later? When does the pendulum swing? Will the baby boomers remain in a bonded contract with their parents' well-being, or are they so preoccupied with their own existences that Ma and Pa are no longer relevant? And what about Ma and Pa? Will they too be so preoccupied with self that endurability of familial tenderness diminishes due to non-use?

Making the Big Location Decision

How do you decide where to spend your last decades? Consider family first, then money, then health, then recreation, and then climate. Where you live your last decades should be an option, not a necessity. During your middle years, work often determines where you live. But when your work is done, the choice of housing locations opens up.

Most people decide to stay close to home. Ninety percent of older persons continue to live in locations near where they lived prior to retirement. A considerable number of older persons who move to the sun upon retirement return to their original cloudier home base. The sense of community you've built over your working years continues to nourish and sustain you even after retirement.

Social experiment and longer life spans have created a new explosion in the variety of housing models available for older people. Every conceivable arrangement is available, from the self-sufficiency of independent living to institutional care in which an individual is tended by a system of organized management. Just where you end up along this spectrum is determined by the core factors listed earlier — family support, finance, health, recreation, and climate, in decreasing order of importance. I am confident that we all would choose the independent end of the scale if we had a choice. No one goes to sleep at night with pleasant anticipation of dependency in the future.

Family considerations

The strength provided by a family convoy is a strong element in maintaining independence. Widowhood is a peril for both sexes. Loss of a spouse is a stern health signal. Having family support nearby can alleviate some of the loneliness and adjustment difficulties after losing a spouse.

Financial considerations

Few people are financially sturdy enough to sustain an unaltered lifestyle after retirement. Usually, people live on a reduced income. For most people, their house is their most valuable asset, and selling it is a temptation. In fact, the 1997 survey revealed that 79 percent of households of persons over the age of 65 were owned by the occupant, and 80 percent of these people owned their homes without a mortgage. The temptation to sell, to cut expenses, and to profit from the increase in real estate values is huge. The negative effect of a house sale, however, is giving up a place you love. You should not take such a decision lightly.

Health considerations

Your functional limitations — if you have any — may be a factor in determining where you live. Commonly, in older people, one of three body functions might be causing limitations — inability to move, inability to control bowels and bladder, and impaired thought processes. Theoretically, none of these problems should prohibit staying home independently, but a functional limitation puts a burden on support systems (such as family). The impact on family must be factored in all decisions.

Climate considerations

Recreation and warm weather are further elements in shaping a decision. Magazines are full of advertisements for retirement communities promising endless golf and shuffleboard and bridge games all played under the benevolent canopy of 75-degree cloudless days. No one can deny the seductiveness of this appeal, but weather is not the most important factor in determining your quality of life, nor should it dominate your decision process about where to live.

Staying in Your Home in Later Years

If the death of spouse, lack of finances, or health problems threaten an older person's independent home existence, an array of options has arisen to assist that person in remaining at home. In some cases, doctors may make house calls to keep the person at home and out of the hospital, for example. Various shared housing arrangements can be made, facilitating cost and security concerns. Taking in a student or other helpful person to assist with chores, or hiring day help, visiting nurses, or meals on wheels, may lighten the care burdens. Local agencies abound that offer helpful suggestions.

One of the most treasured aspects of my professional career has been the privilege of making house calls — and I have made thousands. House calls are part of good medical care. Not only are patients and their families very appreciative, but house calls reduce the need for hospitalization and nursing homes.

For example, immobility and disruptive behavior are more easily addressed at home than after an expensive ambulance ride to a clinic or emergency room. In the case of terminally ill persons, many can remain at home in their last months and days if house calls are still available. And if a home caregiver is present, a house call enables a doctor to make an on-site review of medication compliance. House calls provide a whole host of understandings that are absent in a typical doctor's office visit. On the other hand, house calls are inappropriate for emergency illnesses or accidents.

In 1983, I was privileged to serve as president of the American Geriatrics Society, the major medical group devoted to the health needs of older citizens. I lobbied hard for increased training for physicians about house calls and support for them. Medical schools, Congress, and the American Association of Retired Persons were all strangely indifferent to providing adequate compensation for physicians who make house calls. Physician training and payment for house calls are still grossly inadequate and penalize any increased commitment to this valuable practice. The American Academy of Home Care Physicians carries on this crusade.

Life Beyond Home: Assisted Living

When social, financial, and health reasons conspire to make staying in your home no longer the best option, you can consider an array of living arrangements. Fortunately, assisted living housing is experiencing a boom.

The term *assisted living* encompasses everything from rental to purchase options, with a range of services from little or no added service (a veritable apartment house model) to a full-scale living arrangement that includes three meals a day, home maintenance, and medical surveillance. This level of assisted living will provide care for all but those in need of around-the-clock nursing care.

Assisted living is an active experiment, and new options are being added all the time. The wonderful thing about assisted living is that older persons, as well as their children, can breathe easier knowing that some oversight and support is available. Cost is a substantial issue, as is the adjustment to common living.

 My mother loved her assisted living arrangement — her days were one big party. Having been raised as one of 12 children, she loved the camaraderie of assisted living. She even made sure that she always left her door open, except when she slept.

Handling the Nursing Home Decision

"Mom and Dad, I promise you'll never have to go to a nursing home. We will always take care of you." This solemn contract has been made millions of times only to undergo wrenching reevaluation when caretaking responsibilities become overwhelming. Taking care of an elderly person can create strain on finances or become increasingly difficult as the person's health declines. If you have lots of money and no substantial health deficit, you have no reason to look for a nursing home. When the family support network is pushed to the brink of its capacity, however, many people must consider a nursing home, despite prior promises.

As I confront families in their crisis moment, my advice includes:

- ✔ Are you sure you have exhausted every option for home care?
- ✔ There is no right or wrong here.
- ✔ This decision is not about emotion. It is about seeking the best solution.
- ✔ The best solution is likely not to be a good one, but the least bad one.

> ✔ The best solution for one person is often the worst for another, so the group's best solution is the one to be pursued.
>
> ✔ Any solution for today will not be a final solution. Circumstances change. So, too, do solutions. Any action taken today can be reconsidered tomorrow or next month. No decision is irretrievable.

Part of the discomfort in making this decision is that everyone must wonder about their own aging ahead. People wonder, "Is this what I can expect for myself?"

Nursing home stats

Forty percent of people over 65 will spend some time in a nursing home. The average length of stay is 19 months. However, most people — 44 percent — spend less than three months. On the other extreme, 10 percent spend more than five years there. Of those admitted, 65 percent die in the nursing home. Of the overall nursing home population, 95 percent exhibit some cognitive impairment, and 54 percent are incontinent of bladder or bowel.

There are 16,000 nursing homes in the United States, 70 percent of which are under private management. Admission is highly age dependent. Less than 5 percent of 60- to 70-year-olds are in nursing homes. Twenty-two percent of those aged 85-plus are. Medicare does not cover nursing home costs when the care is deemed "custodial" in nature. Only acute care is reimbursed (for example, after a hip fracture or stroke), and then only for restricted periods. The Medicaid program makes most nursing home payments. To be eligible, you must provide proof of diminished assets and income; many people reshuffle family assets to make sure that they can be eligible. Most nursing homes cost $40,000 per year and up, an amount that exceeds most older persons' budgets.

Checking out the quality of care

Recognizing that the quality of care in nursing homes was a stern problem, sets of guidelines were passed in 1987 about the rights of nursing home residents to self-determination. Before these guidelines, nursing homes were under a substantial threat if any patients died, lest this be determined to be a result of neglect. This resulted in innumerable cruel and improper transfers of dying nursing home residents to hospitals merely to escape administrative review. I have participated in a handful of ugly end-of-life care issues that ended up alienating everyone, because the nursing home was not accepted as a place to die. Now most nursing home residents and their families stipulate their resuscitation wishes in advance, simplifying end-of-life decisions.

In nursing homes, the principal caregivers are nurse's aids. Nurses and nurse's aids in nursing homes are among the world's foremost heroes. Their jobs involve the daily grind of providing knowing, caring, personal services to persons who are often unaware and therefore unappreciative of their services. Not only that, but they must survive in the often hostile environment of the nursing home under a constant threat of regulatory review and penalty. Just the fact that these heroes get out of bed each morning to pursue their life work at sparse wages and with rare thanks makes me grateful for these special caregivers.

Coping with Alzheimer's disease

If it weren't for Alzheimer's disease, we could close almost every nursing home in this country and feel good about it. Today, most patients in nursing homes have Alzheimer's disease. This terrible disease is the main reason people have negative ideas about growing old. Why would I, or anyone, hold any positive hope for my future decades if they were distorted by the multiple indignities imposed by Alzheimer's disease?

Fifty percent of persons over 85 have evidence of Alzheimer's disease, but 50 percent don't. Alzheimer's disease is not a normal part of aging; it is a disease whose cause remains unknown. In only a small percentage of cases is Alzheimer's disease hereditary.

Treatment for the disease is poor. This dreary prospect is partially offset however by rapid advances in the basic science insights about Alzheimer's disease. Hopefully, this core knowledge may yield clues to more effective treatments, or even better, the prevention of the disease.

End-of-Life Care

The brain numbing effect of Alzheimer's disease prompts tough questions: When is life no longer worth living? When is it okay to die? Do we die when the heart stops beating, or when the brain stops knowing? What if the heart keeps beating but the brain is dead? Is that a natural death?

Ethicists agree that even though the heart keeps beating, life is at its logical conclusion when the brain no longer senses. This is a powerful moral stance that immediately raises other issues. What are the criteria for non-sensing — a deep coma, or not being able to recognize family, or inability to speak or move? These questions take us down a slippery slope.

I've staked out my stance on that slippery slope and believe that there are two criteria for non-sensing. First is the inability to perform any functional, life-sustaining activities, such as drinking a glass of water.

Second is the inability to experience joy. My joy test is this: Could the person recognize or react to his grandchildren bounding in Christmas morning to the tree and its goodies? If a person is no longer able to recognize or react to this sort of a basic life experience, then life to me is at its appropriate conclusion.

How long should a person who is brain dead remain on life support? If a person sustains an accident or stroke and is in a coma or is severely lacking in awareness (no joy or function), there may be a possibility that they will recover. Nature sometimes restores people to health, but nature has its limits. One month is currently considered an appropriate period to hope for recovery after a brain catastrophe. If no brain activity has occurred in a month, I believe supporting measures should be withdrawn. This is my personal belief, not official or certified in any way, and I provide it only as a guideline for any of you who may confront this grim situation.

More frequent than the acute event is the gradual loss of cognitive capacity. I have seen hundreds of older persons with advanced Alzheimer's disease lying numbly in nursing homes, unable to move or even swallow. In my view, supplying feeding tubes and the like in this situation is not prolonging life. It is prolonging dying. In my view, if a person can no longer eat, even if fed, then that represents a logical terminus. I have written before that for me an ideal death is one in which there is no pain, tubes, or loneliness. Inserting a feeding tube to a brain dead person, to me, is illogical and wrong.

Understanding the role of a hospice

The hospice movement believes that the process of dying needs to be demedicalized and demystified and returned to its natural state of a valued stage in this process called life. Death is seen not as a disease to be cured, or even dreaded, but as a shared mutual destiny that should be made human again.

The first hospice in the United States opened in Connecticut in 1974. Now there are over 2,000 hospices in the country. Sixty-five percent of hospice patients have cancer. Another 10 percent have cardiovascular disease. The costs of hospice care are covered, in the United States, by private insurance, Medicaid in most states, and Medicare, which means that there are qualifying guidelines. Central to these is the certification, by a physician, that the recipient of hospice care has less than six months to live. Acknowledging the notorious inexpertness of physicians in predicting the timing of death, this issue is ticklish, but we try to fulfill this guideline as best we can.

Hospice care is for treating symptoms, not disease. Hospice caregivers see the person as a whole — physical, emotional, social, and spiritual — and not just as the parts such as the liver, heart, or kidneys. Although hospices have a medical director, nursing is the main hospice process.

Hospice nurses are wonderful friends of dying — they look into its face and know its heart. They comfort always. Elizabeth Kubler Ross formulated the notion that the person engaged in the process of dying traverses five stages — denial, anger, negotiation, depression, and acceptance. Hospice nurses are gentle guides and are wonderful stagehands for the final curtain. Hospice is not just for the patients but for the entire family. Many hospices follow the family for one year after the patient's death.

Choosing how and where to die

You should be in charge of how you die. Much of dying's dread is the notion that the process will be like a freefall, out of control, with no handholds to grasp. This should *never* be the case. Everyone around a dying person is responsible for making sure that the act of dying is in the control of the dying person. That person (who is every one of us) has the solemn obligation to arrange his or her own dying by setting out guidelines.

Very few people have taken the initiative to control their own dying because it seems complicated and awful — but it needn't be. For starters, I suggest this testament: "I hereby assert that when my end is at hand, I wish to have no pain, no tubes, and be at home with those I love. Further, I wish my ending to be short, simple, and convenient. If this means increasing the doses of medication to ensure ease and dignity, I authorize and encourage their use."

Make this declaration to a responsible loved one at any appropriate life moment — a quiet, relaxed moment when everyone is at ease. You don't have to be sick or very old to talk about this issue. Don't wait until the bitter end, because you need to deliver the statement with clarity and lack of emotion — both of which are hard to do when you are near death.

Living wills and advanced directives are more standard and formalized instructions about the dying act. You may also assign durable power of attorney for healthcare. The specifics of these legal documents in the United States vary from state to state, and you need to track them. In my experience with several thousand patients, the presence or absence of a formal document, though helpful, is not nearly as important as the solemn agreement my patient and I have made about the person's desire to control the dying process. I merely act as the person's agent. Patients, physicians, and family members must communicate about the covenant. Dying loses its sting when the dying person remains in charge until the final breath is taken.

Part III
Handling a Health Crisis

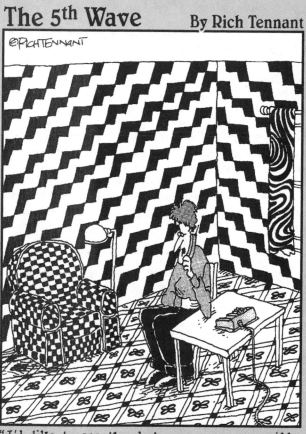

"I'd like to see the doctor as soon as possible. The nausea, dizziness, and disorientation just seem to persist day after day."

In this part . . .

As we age, our chances of being involved in an emergency health situation increase. That prospect can be unsettling, but, however suddenly those situations arise, there are ways to be prepared. Chapter 11 shows you what to expect in an emergency. From what signs indicate that it's time to go to the emergency room to getting to the hospital, this chapter prepares you for what you can expect during an emergency room visit. If a hospital stay is necessary, Chapter 12 shows you how to make the most out of your time spent in a health institution. And, if surgery is a possibility, look to Chapter 13 for information on making surgical decisions with your physician, understanding how aging affects surgery, and choosing the right surgeon.

Chapter 11

Understanding Your Role in an Emergency Situation

- -

In This Chapter

▶ Knowing when an emergency is an emergency

▶ Learning what to do, step by step, in an emergency

▶ Discovering the ins and outs of the emergency system

▶ Taking charge in a moment of crisis

- -

*I*f you're doing your best to stay healthy, you're learning the mindset and strategies that can help you stay out of the sickness system. In reality, however, sometimes even the best-laid plans don't work out, and you may need outside help — which is where the emergency system comes in.

Your primary care doctor is your first line of recourse (see Chapter 2 for more on the importance of this doctor). Emergencies such as accidents and acute (sudden) illness are much less common among older people than chronic (lingering) illness — 70 to 80 percent of the illnesses of older persons are chronic in nature. Nevertheless, older people are not immune to emergency situations, so you should prepare yourself as best you can for such a possibility.

An emergency can be anything from a nosebleed that won't stop to unexplained loss of memory. An emergency is anything that elicits sufficient alarm that if something isn't done quickly the situation might get plenty worse.

This chapter explains how you and your acute response system should work. It covers both the "wheres" and the "whys." The first lesson is being sure you know the wheres — the telephone number of your doctor, the number of the emergency room in your hospital, and, of course, 911 (which is pretty well etched into everyone's mental telephone book).

After you have secured your where information, the why questions arise — why should you go to an emergency room? This chapter outlines the big worry emergencies and some of the major symptoms that cause concern. It gives a brief course in the use of medicine, hospitals, and surgeons. These three wonderful resources provide security when you need them, but you must first know how to access them to best benefit from their rescuing efforts.

First Things First: Your Primary Care Physician's Role

Acute illness and injuries are the main business of the emergency room (ER). When a major acute problem appears, no single advice can tell you whether you should call your doctor first, call 911, or go directly to the ER. You should discuss this potential scenario the first time you meet your doctor. The best scenario would find your primary care doctor otherwise non-occupied and able personally to attend to your emergency needs. If your doctor is immediately available to receive your urgent call, you'll lose no time before the next step is initiated if hospitalization is called for. If, however, you can't reach your doctor immediately, you need to enter the emergency system on your own.

The big advantage to informing your physician before your visit to the ER, is that your doctor can supply important background information to the ER staff. Your primary care doc is also able to mobilize the reports and services of specialist doctors who may have played some past role in your medical history. Several studies have shown that the outcome of ER visits is improved when the primary care doctor is involved in the care management. This same benefit of sustained participation of your primary doctor is confirmed at every level of hospital care up to and including the intensive care unit, and beyond. Encourage your doctor to visit you in the hospital or in the emergency room. The hospital is a daunting place, and the familiarity you have achieved with your basic physician is strong therapy, whatever your problem is.

Deciding If It's an Emergency or Not

Older people use the emergency room a lot. In 1998 there were over 100 million visits to the ER. About one-third of these were because of injuries. In 1998, there were over 15 million visits to the ER by persons over 65 years of age, and evidence suggests that when people reach 75 years of age and older, the number of visits increases.

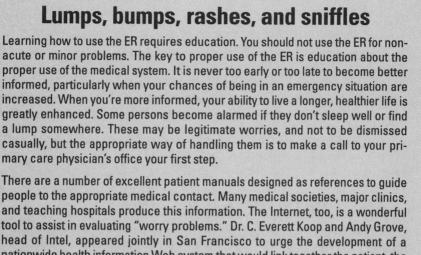

Lumps, bumps, rashes, and sniffles

Learning how to use the ER requires education. You should not use the ER for non-acute or minor problems. The key to proper use of the ER is education about the proper use of the medical system. It is never too early or too late to become better informed, particularly when your chances of being in an emergency situation are increased. When you're more informed, your ability to live a longer, healthier life is greatly enhanced. Some persons become alarmed if they don't sleep well or find a lump somewhere. These may be legitimate worries, and not to be dismissed casually, but the appropriate way of handling them is to make a call to your primary care physician's office your first step.

There are a number of excellent patient manuals designed as references to guide people to the appropriate medical contact. Many medical societies, major clinics, and teaching hospitals produce this information. The Internet, too, is a wonderful tool to assist in evaluating "worry problems." Dr. C. Everett Koop and Andy Grove, head of Intel, appeared jointly in San Francisco to urge the development of a nationwide health information Web system that would link together the patient, the physician, and the healthcare organizations to facilitate quick medical information exchange whenever it is required. Such a system is sure to come because its value and cost effectiveness are self-evident.

WebMD (www.webmd.com) and CBShealthwatch (www.cbshealthwatch.com) are reliable Web sites to which you can refer for more information.

Some individuals use the emergency room inappropriately for conditions that do not really qualify as emergencies. The ER should not substitute for the doctor's office or clinic. For most conditions, just because your doctor doesn't have an immediate appointment available, doesn't mean you should head directly to the emergency room.

It's an emergency when...

What are the important signs to signal an emergency? When do you send up a distress flare? When do you require immediate emergency care? Certain major symptoms are clear situations that demand emergency attention, for example:

- ✔ Lack of breathing or pulse
- ✔ Unconsciousness
- ✔ Major change in mental state (confusion, drowsiness, and so forth)
- ✔ Active major bleeding
- ✔ Shortness of breath at rest

✔ Severe pain

✔ Major injury

✔ Ingestion of excessive medications or other toxic substances

✔ Inability to urinate or have a bowel movement

Every one of these red flares indicates that one or more life-threatening events have occurred. Loss of consciousness could mean stroke, or poisoning, or shock, or a diabetic coma. Pain accompanies injury, or blockage of anything, or heart attack, or childbirth. Major symptoms demand major attention, and the ER is usually the place where the diagnosis is made and treatment started.

Getting to the ER on time

Of the hundreds of potential emergency conditions, only a relatively few are truly time-critical. The brain can withstand only a few minutes without adequate blood supply. The heart's reserve capacity is similarly measured only in minutes before major damage results from a blocked artery. When a heart attack is suspected, you need help — ASAP.

Your own individual circumstances dictate whether you should use personal transportation to head to the ER or the ambulance. The ambulance takes time to reach you, from just a few minutes to much longer, depending on where you live. This inevitable delay should be balanced against the immediate help that the paramedics are available to provide on the spot when they arrive. Paramedics are generally well-trained professionals with 1,000 hours of training in procedures to be employed in acute situations. Elective defibrillation, intravenous fluid and medication initiation, oxygen, and CPR are some of their tools that, on occasion, can save your life. Paramedics usually are in direct phone contact with the emergency room, where a physician can receive the initial condition report, and provide stopgap treatment advisories before the ambulance reaches the ER.

Early response has been so effective that many at-risk people are using home monitoring devices. A person with a heart rhythm irregularity, for example, can be hooked up by radio to a central locale that alerts a system to a possible problem. Half of the heart attack fatalities occur before a doctor or a paramedic can be summoned — and a heart attack occurs in the United States every 20 seconds. That's a lot of people who are dying before help can arrive. Clearly, any ability for earlier awareness should have huge payoffs. Already, a proportion of the decreased number of deaths from heart attacks is due to better informed and effective emergency response procedures.

Almost always, insurance covers emergency situations, even if you encounter such a situation out of the country. Problems only arise when the visit is deemed not to be an emergency, as it first appeared. This is when negotiations start. Your primary physician may be asked to provide documentation, which will assist in any negotiating that might occur.

The big reasons for visiting the ER

The main reasons you may find yourself in the ER include heart attacks, pain, behavior changes, injuries, bleeding, overdoses, and problems with vital signs and bodily output. This section takes a look at some of the possible symptoms of problems in those areas, and shows you what your doctor will be doing to treat those problems in the ER.

Saying, "Don't panic," is easy, but actually staying calm is sometimes hard to do. I have witnessed seasoned medical doctors losing their cool when a family member was endangered. The best protection against this panic is preparation. Rehearse what you might do in case of a fall or other misadventure. Know the phone number you would need to call, or have the number available. One trick is to post a list of your medicines in a prominent place in your home, such as on the refrigerator, where the paramedics might discover it if you became unconscious. Although slower than going directly to the ER by car, calling 911 brings trained professionals who know how to assess and initiate in-the-field treatment.

Is it a heart attack?

A heart attack looms largest of all the acute situations, simply because it is the number one killer in the Western World. Everyone should be aware of the symptoms of a heart attack so they can act as their own emergency cardiologist.

Heart pain is most commonly crushing — like an elephant's foot stepping on you. The pain can occur anywhere between the earlobe and the belly button, but is most frequently encountered beneath the breastbone. If you note shortness of breath, weakness, dizziness, sweating, or an irregular pulse beat, don't waste any time in calling for help. If you are having a heart attack and these symptoms are not present, there is a very good chance you will be okay. Only a quarter of persons who consult the emergency room with chest pain actually turn out to have suffered damage to the heart muscle. There are hosts of other non-heart causes of chest pain that your health system is practiced at evaluating. Relaxation and two aspirins are good advice for many situations, and they also have been shown to be strong remedies for the person who actually is having a heart attack. However, you should still go to the ER if heart attack symptoms arise.

As a young doctor, I recall receiving streams of healthy young men with chest pain, which they thought was due to their heart. Simply pressing on their ribs provoked the same pain, which ruled out heart disease. Almost all of these men were smokers, and their repeated hacking cough irritated the cartilage of the chest wall and provoked the pain. Hopefully, most of these guys gave up the habit after this scare.

A heart attack occurs when one of the three small arteries that supply the heart itself with blood becomes clogged with a clot or a clump of cholesterol. A heart attack may or may not be associated with a bout of exercise. Depending on its location, the blockage deprives part of the heart of its blood, similar to what happens when you apply a tourniquet to your finger, including the throbbing and hurting. If a blockage can be relieved early enough, damage to the heart can be limited or prevented entirely. The severity of the injury can often be judged by the corresponding symptoms. The most worrisome symptoms are a fall in blood pressure, shortness of breath, and an irregularity of the heart beat.

This is the nuts and bolts of a heart attack, but, as often happens in life, a major exception exists. Older people are notorious for not following the rules of heart attack symptoms. Whereas "crushing, sub-sternal chest pain" is the standard description of a heart attack pain, older people may complain only of light-headedness, fatigue, or shortness of breath — which are symptoms commonly associated with a damaged heart muscle. (In fact, for decades, heart trouble was usually passed off as "acute indigestion." Before 1950, hundreds of thousands of persons died of heart attacks but with the wrong diagnosis stuck on them.) As a result of this unreliability and variability of the symptom pattern of older persons, your primary care doctor would be well-advised to take an extra step or two in the diagnostic survey just to make sure that this important diagnosis is not overlooked.

Identifying dangerous changes in behavior

When a person loses consciousness or shows a marked alteration in behavior, such as frenzy or stupor, then you have an emergency. The causes for such an alarming symptom vary from injury to poisoning to strokes to diabetes and more. In such cases, emergency personnel will focus all initial efforts on ensuring that the person survives, and, after the person's condition is stabilized, the doctor can pursue the search for the underlying cause.

All available information needs to be gathered. Empty pills bottles? Alcohol? A fall? Prior illness? Then the physical exam is conducted. Temperature, blood pressure, and pulse are taken and respiratory abnormalities are detected. Whether one side of the body or both is involved is critical. Disparity in pupil size? Neck stiffness? Then laboratory tests are initiated on the blood, urine, spinal fluid, and x-rays so that, hopefully, an explanatory diagnosis is established in the shortest time possible. Even strokes, previously dismal in their prognosis, are becoming susceptible to successful treatment, particularly if the treatment is begun promptly.

Injuries that demand attention

How doctors handle situations in which a major injury has occurred (for example, due to a fall or a motor vehicle accident) depends on the symptoms experienced by the patient. If there is any hint of injury to the head, spinal cord, or chest, then immediate measures are called for — those areas are where really acute problems reside. If any of these situations prevail, then all stops are pulled out to address the life or major body functioning problem. However, if a person is conscious and can move and breathe, then the situation is less alarming.

Falls are a frequent and insistent emergency problem of older persons. My advice to my healthy 95-year-old mother was "don't fall down." She fell down at least two times in her mid-90s, breaking her wrist. But, she insisted on wearing medium heels on her shoes. (Vanity is present even in 90-year-olds!) Still, because she was 50 pounds overweight, she was padded somewhat against hip fractures, and she was strong. Consequently, her falls cost her, but not a lot. Other older people are not so lucky, and falls are a major cause of death in old people.

Never neglect a fall. The older body is more fragile, and despite the bother of an emergency room visit, it is far better to be safe than sorry. Falls can kill, if not acutely, then chronically, if they are neglected. Early injury treatment generally means as short a time in bed as possible.

Urination or bowel movement problems

When we think of emergencies, we tend to think of intake problems — the inability to breath, swallow, or drink, for example. However, output problems with urination or having a bowel movement are more common in older persons than input problems. Urinary or bowel obstructions are regular alarms that send older persons to the emergency room because there are no home remedies for urinary or colon obstruction.

Problems with urinary flow are far more common in males than females because of that troublesome little prostate gland. This lime-sized organ, which lies deeply hidden in our pelvis, occupies a critical anatomic site where the urethra empties the bladder. Very commonly, this gland become enlarged and narrows the outflow. Some drugs, including commonly used antihistamines, can aggravate the situation. Only a little additional swelling needs to occur before the prostate totally shuts off the flow of urine from the bladder. This is very distressing, and requires immediate attention, as acute urinary retention is extremely unpleasant.

In a similar way, the intestines must empty themselves on a regular basis. If they don't, waste materials plug up the flow and an intestinal obstruction occurs. Like urinary retention, intestinal obstruction is an emergency situation. Abdominal distention and discomfort, nausea, vomiting, and collapse follow. The most common causes of blocked intestines in older people are adhesions from previous surgery and fecal impaction (which results from failure of the normal passage of fecal material and its consequent hardening and blocking). Using laxatives and enemas, medical personnel will try to dislodge the blockage. Often, however, such blockages require physical removal by hand or tube. Sometimes a blockage can require surgery, depending on the cause.

Bleeding problems

Bleeding comes in various forms. Most bleeding problems are minor, but some are major. A nosebleed, for example, is usually a minor problem. If the nosebleed is profuse and prolonged, however, it can become an emergency — and I have tended many of these in the ER.

When bleeding is external, evaluation is pretty easy. Internal bleeding, on the other hand, creates greater worry. One indication of internal bleeding is vomiting of blood, which may signal an ulcer or a tumor. However, most internal bleeding is identifiable by a change in color of the bowel movement. A bright red bowel movement indicates a bleeding source near the rectum. A black, tarry bowel movement indicates a problem further upstream. The critical issue confronted in the emergency room with gastrointestinal bleeding is the pace of the bleeding. How much and how fast is the bleeding point leaking? The blood pressure and pulse rate are first-line indicators. A rapid pulse and low blood pressure means something must be done right away. The blood tests repeated at timed intervals also give an idea of how fast the leak is proceeding and what degree of urgency is appropriate. One of the most common causes of gastrointestinal bleeding is anti-inflammatory medications consumed by millions of arthritis sufferers. These drugs all carry the hazard of irritation of the stomach and intestine, and the first evidence of this is often a black bowel movement.

Overdoses of medication

Overdoses of medications or other toxins, accidental or otherwise, are also the everyday business of the emergency room. In this situation, medical history is critical, because the search for the cause of an unexplained poisoning is hazardous and complex. Identification of the offending substance is vital.

If you suspect someone has been poisoned, here's what you can do to help: If the person is unconscious, summon help immediately. If the person is conscious and if the nature of the poisoning is a strong acid, alkali, or oil (such as paint remover, harsh cleaners, or weed killers), give him or her milk or milk of magnesia. If the suspected poison is a medicine, try to induce vomiting by putting your finger down the back of the patient's throat or by administering 2 tablespoons of syrup of ipecac. The number of your local poison control center, if not the same as your hospital ER, should be on your "being prepared" roster — along with the numbers of your doctor, dentist, pharmacist, paramedics, and hospital — and a quick call is certainly in order.

Navigating the ER Successfully

The emergency room tends to be a scary place — it is certainly not like home. With its bright lights and shining surfaces, urgent commands, and strange smells, the ER is disorienting, and not at all conducive to easing anxiety. If you aren't prepared for what you'll encounter in the ER, anxiety can definitely result.

If you find yourself in the ER, access to information can help remedy your anxiety. If the attending physician and staff is able to provide you with knowledge of what is going on and how long you will be in the ER, then you get some sense of reassurance and confidence. Given all the increased testing that now goes on, stays of many hours in the ER are not uncommon, and the tedium and uncertainties are taxing for everyone. If your primary care physician has been playing a guiding, coordinating, and informing role in all that is going on, you will be in good hands. That is the ideal.

If a patient has end-of-life directives, a primary care doctor should relay that information to the emergency room staff. When a patient rolls through the ER doors with no blood pressure, pulse, or respiration, the ER staff knows what to do. However, the staff shouldn't pull out all the stops if the person has already indicated that heroic measures (usually meaning insertion of life-sustaining tubes) are not wanted. Without prompt availability of this information, the staff proceeds immediately to restore the vital functions. I have been witness to dozens of situations in which tubes were inserted almost in a reflex manner, because no advisory accompanied the person. When the information arrives, minutes or hours later, the tubes are already in place. Withdrawing them, while easily accomplished, still represents an effort that would have been better avoided than remedied after the fact, thereby sparing indignity, discomfort, and cost.

Identifying your pain

Pain is Mother Nature's distress signal. Pain lets you know that something is wrong. In terms of sheer numbers, arthritis and back pain are the most common reasons for pain, but they rarely qualify as a reason to seek emergency care.

If you're a patient in the ER, your doctor or nurse might ask you to describe pain in terms of when it happens, what produces it, and what relieves it. In addition, you will be asked to describe the intensity on a scale of one to ten — ten being absolutely unbearable, shrieking pain, and one as a minor nagging ache. This numerical rating of the pain helps your doctor understand the severity of the situation. Of course, one-to-ten is not a perfect rule, because some pretty minor issues such as shingles can hurt like hell, while other major conditions, such as appendicitis, may be rather low in their pain rating. Considerable competence is required to evaluate pain. Pain always means that a problem exists — the issue is simply finding out the source of the problem so that you can undertake appropriate treatment.

The duration of the pain is also of consequence. Any abrupt, severe pain demands immediate attention. If pain is less acute and comes and goes, there is generally some grace period in evaluating it, but the whole pain area demands careful vigilance before assigning a low worry score to it.

As with other major symptoms, pain is more serious in the older people than in younger people, because they generally have diminished reserves of strength, and it helps to be physically strong if a pain hits. Treatment of pain, of course, depends on the cause, but continued pain needs to be addressed promptly when it occurs.

Paying attention to vital signs

Pulse rate, temperature, blood pressure, and respiratory rate are called "vital signs" in medical lingo, because they represent how the basic body functions are working. Your vital signs will be checked regularly if you have to visit the ER. Generally, each vital sign is maintained within a fairly narrow range. Whenever any of these exceed these tolerable values, a problem exists. Occasionally the signs by themselves indicate a big problem. If the pulse is above 150 or below 40, that's bad. Similarly, if the blood pressure, temperature, or respiratory rate is unacceptably high or low, an emergency may be at hand. Already available are very serviceable home monitors that track these four basic functions. The time is not far off when a person, who has been judged to be at risk of a condition where problems may be heralded by a jump up or fall off of one of these measurements, can have an early detection system in place.

Normal Ranges for Bodily Functions

Pulse	45–80 per minute
Respiration	8–20 per minute
Temperature	97–99.5(°F)
Blood pressure	130/85–90/60 mmHg

Using the Urgent Care Center as an In Between Step

Let's face it: the medical system has its negative points, including the all-too-common problem of long waits for routine doctor appointments, and inappropriate use of the emergency room for non-emergency purposes. Fortunately, a new entity has sprung up so that if your ailment doesn't fall into the categories described earlier, you don't have to wait for medical attention. The urgent care center (UCC) is meant to bridge the gap between your doctor's office and the emergency room. We didn't have UCC's when I was a young doctor, but things were simpler then. Doctors had more time, and ERs weren't overwhelming and frightfully expensive.

The UCC has appeared to fill an interim need for persons with problems that are severe enough to warrant a doctor evaluation sooner than your primary care has an available free slot, but not severe enough to warrant the intensity of the emergency room. My community has several urgent care centers available, staffed by qualified persons and capable of performing a whole set of interim diagnostic evaluations and treatments. Sometimes the UCC will recognize that hospital care is appropriate and transfer the patient. Usually, however, the staff will refer the patient back to the primary care doctor for follow-up. As with emergency room encounters, your primary care physician should know of your visit to the UCC and make your current records available.

The UCCs are wonderful — they serve to defuse the time bind between your primary care doctor and the hospital. But UCCs do have limits. The staff and care are non-continuous. In other words, the UCC is not intended to provide continuity of care, but is devoted to specific problems that the other parts of your medical care system are temporarily incapable of handling. You can think of a UCC as a triage center, capable of early evaluation and minor treatments, but it serves primarily as a stopgap entity.

UCCs are utilized most commonly after hours or over weekends. They are also valuable if a non-emergency illness hits when you are away from home without a physician contact. You should think of them as a stopgap convenience, filling a temporary need. As with ER use, insurance coverage for a UCC visit is generally available, providing the indications for the visit are reasonable. Occasionally, an authorizing phone call to the insurance office is involved.

Chapter 12

Making the Hospital Work for You

● ●

In This Chapter
▶ Treating aging patients
▶ Receiving the best hospital care

● ●

*N*o one relishes the prospect of a trip to the hospital, yet we are immensely happy that the hospital is there for us in time of need. In many communities, the hospital is one of our most cherished and respected resources. Many of us share a loyalty to our local hospital, as we do to our primary care doctor. The hospital is potentially a very important ally in our healthcare, and it's important to get familiar with the hospital and its workings.

The New Hospital in the New Millennium

The institution we know as the hospital is constantly reviewing itself and making changes. Once a dreary home for the dying and incurable, the hospital has transformed itself into a center of technological miracles. Changes occur with a startling rapidity. The hospital my father practiced in just 50 years ago bears little resemblance to the hospital of today.

If you think hospitals can be somewhat frightening places today, be glad you weren't in a hospital in 1910. That year, a report on the state of medical care in the United States found broad deficiencies in hospitals. As a result, 60 percent of the nation's hospitals were closed down!

Formerly, all three phases of an illness (diagnosis, treatment, and recuperation) took place in the hospital. Any obscure complaint prompted admission to the hospital so the problem could be sorted out, diagnosed, treated, and recovered from. Now, only the treatment phase of the illness takes place within the hospital. Usually the diagnosis has been established before entering into the sanitized walls of the hospital, and recuperation is shifted to less costly sites.

Cost issues have driven the shift in the role of the hospital. Today, the hospital is the epitome of a time-crunching machine, a place driven insistently by the immense increase in the cost of a hospital stay. The cost of the typical hospital bed used to be 100 dollars a day when I graduated from medical school in 1955. Today, that amount will buy you only an hour or two in most hospitals.

The incredible shrinking length of stay

Not too many decades ago, patients were admitted into the hospital for every possible medical issue, including weight loss programs. Heart attack victims commonly stayed in the hospital for over a month. A bad back often resulted in a prescription for two weeks in bed in the hospital. These long-term stays kept hospitals full. In contrast, last year I participated in the care of a patient with severe diabetes plus complications who underwent a pancreas and kidney transplant, a drama of surreal immensity. Sicknesses don't get more savage than his. Operations don't get more heroic than his. Amazingly, this patient was discharged from the hospital six days after entry.

Today's hospitals can be considered an enlarged intensive care unit. Almost all patients in the hospital now are very sick and require the most complex, sophisticated, labor-intensive effort to tend their needs. Fancy machines with fancier technologists crowd the work floors. Hospital bills of several thousand dollars a day are common — and that's before the doctor submits a fee.

Why the dramatic shift in length of stay? Back in the 1980s, policy makers became acutely aware of the increase in hospital costs and crafted a host of major laws designed to modulate the escalation of hospital expense. Among these changes was the introduction of payment to the hospital not for the number of days spent in the hospital, but rather by specific diagnosis. This policy shift had two important results: shorter stays became a big incentive for hospitals, and hospital administrators learned how to maximize payments to the hospital by creative diagnostic coding.

Unfortunately, neither of these changes benefited the patient. In fact, the phrase "quicker and sicker" (meaning that hospitals were anxious to discharge patients earlier, thereby closer to their initial emergency encounter) became common. Great alarm was sounded about premature discharges from the hospital. Stability was assured by the hiring of "discharge planners," whose job was to be aware of the patient shortly after admission, track the hospital course, and be prepared to offer prompt post-discharge alternative care circumstances when the acute problem had been addressed.

Because of this influence, lengths of stay in the hospital shortened dramatically. Further, new entities have been created such as surgecenters and home management strategies that allowed procedures, including many surgeries, to be performed without even going to the hospital. Now procedures that formerly would have meant at least several days in the hospital are done on an outpatient basis.

There has been much public attention given to what is known as "drive through deliveries." My wife was in the hospital for 13 days with our firstborn child and only three days for our fourth child — and that was 40 years ago. At that rate, I wonder if she would even be in the hospital at all these days!

While shortened hospital stays have slowed the increase in national hospital costs — a good thing — they have also resulted in the closure of many hospitals — not always a good thing. Many hospitals whose decreased numbers of "bed days" were insufficient for their survival ended up out of business, many in rural areas. Certainly no one would recommend having more hospitals than we need, but rural residents have suffered from the decreased availability of convenient hospital care.

The downside of hospitals

Hospitals are sources of miracles. They are also sources of miseries. Several probing studies have recently detailed the high amount of mischief that goes on within hospital walls. Some of this is carelessness, some neglect, some incompetence, and almost none is intentional. The point remains, however, that hospitals can be dangerous, particularly for older persons with diminished coping capacities.

There are 180,000 deaths in hospitals caused by the medical system each year. (That's more than three times the number of U.S. soldiers killed in Vietnam!) Another 1.3 million are injured. The sicker a person is, the greater are the chances for harm. Not only are the body's reserves less, but more dangerous procedures and treatments are performed in a desperate effort to help. Ironically, some critics have said that hospitals have become as dangerous today as they were in the "bad old days" before we knew or could do anything for our sickest.

One survey found that one-quarter of older hospital patients develop confusion in the hospital. Confusion compounds risk, as our "antennae" are blunted. Unfortunately, nutritional needs are sometimes neglected during the acute stages of the hospital encounter, further weakening an already burdened system. Of even greater concern is the lack of physical activity during a hospital stay. Going to bed is dangerous in its own right, and the added debility created when a person is on his or her back for prolonged periods of time compromises recovery. In fact, enforced inactivity leads to a loss of muscle strength of

2 percent per day. At that rate, you could calculate that a week in bed is a serious health threat — and more than a week can be disastrous all by itself.

A colleague, Dr. Calvin Hirsch, conducted a survey of the functional capacity of patients when they leave the hospital compared with that when they entered the hospital. He found that they were worse off, often much worse off, by the time they went home. This worsening was due largely to the decline caused by bed rest.

Bedsores are an ugly but common result of hospitalization that involves prolonged bed rest. I have cared for hundreds of patients with bedsores, which are basically preventable and always an embarrassment. A bed sore occurs at a pressure point (tail bone, heels, shoulder blades, and so forth) when that part of the body has been allowed to remain for long periods without pressure relief. When a lot of things are going on with a hospitalized patient, as they always are, and with many other more pressing concerns, it is simply too easy to neglect shifting the posture to relieve pressure. A pressure sore can start to occur within one day, so regular vigilance is necessary. If a person has diminished awareness, either because of the medical condition itself or because of medications, the risk of a bedsore goes way up.

Aging Patients in the Hospital

I feel strongly that age should rarely, if ever, be used as a criterion for whether or not a person can use the hospital — or anything else, for that matter. Such a policy leads to innumerable bad decisions. I recall inheriting the medical care of a fine 98-year-old woman upon the retirement of a colleague. This woman had a steady bleeding from her bladder, and her former doctor had presumed that it was likely due to some unremediable condition and chose not to pursue it. Because of this bleeding, she was chronically anemic and fatigued. I felt otherwise and arranged for a urologist to look into her bladder with an instrument under anesthesia. What was found was a small polyp that was actually bleeding, and was easily removed. The bleeding stopped, the anemia reversed, and the quality of her life improved dramatically.

In my first book, _We Live Too Short and Die Too Long,_ I recall my decision to continue the intensive treatment of an 85-year-old woman suffering from a "flail chest," which resulted from a very aggressive resuscitation effort. After weeks of heroic care she went home, lived an excellent additional year with her husband and then died acutely at home. The bill for intensive treatment was $85,000, totally paid for by Medicare. In effect, a healthy and happy year of life for an 85-year-old woman was bought for $85,000. Some ethicists could argue that I should have let her die in the intensive care unit, because spending that much money on an 85-year-old was immoral. I disagree. If her life quality had been different, I would have advised accordingly, but as long as I knew she had the potential for functional recovery I felt that pulling out all the stops was appropriate, even though she was old.

Age is an inappropriate marker for important medical decisions. Much more important than age in deciding who should receive what treatment is the quality of life of the person at risk. Some people in their 30s should not receive high-cost hospital care because of diminished functional quality of life, in my opinion. Some people in their 90s and beyond should receive intensive, expensive treatment because the potential still exists for healthy added years. To make these decisions on the basis of age alone is morally wrong.

In a study at the Stanford Hospital Intensive Care Unit a few years ago, then medical student Bill Sage and I looked at the results of the experiences of old people there. When all other conditions were standardized, we found that age alone did not predict good or bad results.

Nationwide statistics indicate that age is being increasingly disregarded as a consideration for hospitalization and intensive care. We can derive pretty accurate predictions of which persons will or will not be likely to benefit from a trip to the hospital using formulas to measure how the heart, brain, kidneys, and lungs are working. By adding up these scores we can come up with a predictive idea of how things are likely to turn out. Age is not on this list, and shouldn't be. Symptoms do not present themselves until only 30 percent of maximum function remains. The older a person is, the greater are the chances that these resources are depleted. But most deficits are reversible, and are not age dependent. A person's age alerts the physician to the potential of decreased reserves, but does not tell how much can be done to restore the loss.

If you are an older prospective patient to a hospital, or the family of such a person, be vigilant that those in charge are approaching crucial decisions using the vital information at hand to guide their actions — and not your age. The question always should be "What can you do?" not "How old are you?"

Taking Charge: An Insider's Guide to a Hospital Stay

Can today's high-speed, complex hospital be taught to be more user-friendly? Certainly, many forces conspire to make it less friendly. Merely the volume and tempo of strange encounters are enough to spook any stoic. A hospital is as unlike home as a subway station or a boiler factory. Is that any place to go to get better? Probably not, but by preparing in advance and taking control of your hospital stay, you will find the hospital a much less threatening environment. Here is what to look for in a hospital, and what to watch for during your stay:

- ✔ The hospital should provide as congenial an environment for creature comforts as possible. Sounds, light, and smell need constant surveillance. Private rooms generally encourage peace. Tranquility encourages healing, while clamor invites deterioration. Beds and furnishings should provide maximum comfort.

- ✔ Use of drugs needs to be scrupulously surveyed. The best drug is the one not administered. The hospital is a source of intensive medication usage, but the opportunity for harm abounds. Any symptoms from headache to diarrhea to unexplained weight loss may signify an adverse drug reaction. Suspicion should always arise when doses are increased or upon addition of an another medication. Some medicines when taken alone may be without hazard, but in combination there is hazard. The best example of this is blood thinners taken with most arthritis medicines, which raises the chance of bleeding considerably.

- ✔ The diagnostic tests need to be critically monitored. The numbers of tests that hospital patients undergo has multiplied exponentially in the past 20 years. Each test, even a blood test, has its risks. In particular, tests that use diagnostic dyes have hazards associated with their use and should be watched carefully.

    Always of concern because of frequent mischief with their use are the dyes used in some x-ray examinations. Any reaction to one of these dyes becomes a vital part of your medical history, which you should always be aware of, even to the extent of wearing a med-alert bracelet telling of this sensitivity.

- ✔ Every directive on a doctor's order sheet should be written with a high sensitivity to the costs associated with that test or treatment. All doctors are guilty of blithely scribbling routine orders out of habit, rather than because of considered necessity. Some institutions provide the costs of tests directly in the ordering area.

    Cost is not something most patients are aware of when doctors prescribe a medicine or order a test. Doctors, however, should all be constantly asking themselves, "Is this order necessary? Does the benefit justify the cost?" Being a good patient means letting your doctor know that you too are a responsible member of the health team, and this means price consciousness too.

- ✔ Never forget the value of exercise. I have often thought that moving the TV set from the foot of the bed to the head, thereby requiring the patient to be out of bed to watch, might be as strong a medicine as one that comes in pill form. I have also advocated the use of physical therapists for most hospital patients, not just those recovering from a stroke or an accident. Every person needs muscles, and these should be in at least as good of condition on discharge from the hospital as on admission, and early and frequent ambulation is one way to achieve this. I have actually advocated recording corridor trips the patient makes each day as a helpful guide to recovery.

✔ Food should be tasteful and attractive. Being in an alien place is bad enough without having to cope with cold or tasteless food. If, as a patient, you develop a craving for a particular food treat, ask your doctor if your family can provide it.

✔ The prospect of a hospital being a foreign country staffed by hosts of strangers is not conducive to good care and good morale. Nurses are crucial to your care and recovery, and the closer you can bond with them the better able they will be in sharing your sickness burden. I encourage you to recognize that your primary care doctor should remain intimately involved with your in-hospital experience, either directly as you attending physician, or in regular contact with that individual and with you. Good communication is good medicine.

✔ Don't tolerate pain. Pain delays recovery, and being "strong" or placid and lying stoically with clenched teeth is not good medical advice. Pain management is growing up as a medical capability, and with diligence and intelligence pain should not be a major burden to recovery.

✔ Encourage visitors. Aside from rare instances such as infectious disease isolation, maintaining the close embrace of family and friends helps healing. Getting well is best accomplished as a group effort, and the estrangement that the older person undergoes because of illness should not be compounded by a lack of social contact.

✔ Plan to get out of the hospital ASAP. Strange as it might seem, some people enjoy being in the hospital. You, however, should have a strategy for keeping your hospital stay as short as possible. That may even involve a conditioning program before entering the hospital, so that muscle strength is good throughout your stay. And returning home doesn't have to be scary. Many arrangements can be made to make your return a positive part of the healing experience. Home health agencies, visiting nurses, meals on wheels, and more are available to assist you.

Don't go home too early. Any new symptom or change in vital sign (a temperature or fast pulse) or instability of any sort should be addressed before leaving the hospital. Get all your questions answered before you leave. The better informed you become about what you can expect when you return home, the better your long-term result will be.

Learning how to use and not to use the hospital is a task that we didn't learn about in grade school. But as we mature, we have the opportunity to learn about these institutions that play important roles in our lives. Don't wait for the siren to sound to learn more about your hospital. Make it your friend, and become comfortable and familiar with it now.

Chapter 13

Surgery and the Older Patient

* *

In This Chapter

▶ Understanding surgery

▶ Choosing a surgeon

▶ Aging and surgery

* *

*O*ftentimes, hospital stays result in surgery. Just as the modern-day hospital is undergoing momentous change, so too is the hospital's major activity — surgery. While most people have an encounter with a surgeon at some time in their lives, usually it's for minor issues such as mole removal or hernia repair. But the truly heroic surgical feats are still the focus of great interest and fascination. Today's surgeon needs to be a highly competent technician, able to use increasingly powerful and expensive new tools.

How do you make good decisions about surgery when confronted with an often intimidating, technological world of surgical options? Read on for some sound advice on surgical decisions.

Big Trends in Surgery

Modern surgery traditionally has treated tumors, injuries, burns, and infections. Today, however, surgery is reaching into reconstructive areas, gene transfer and engineering, and tissue and organ transplantation. Science fiction and surgery are sometimes hard to distinguish when we read of artificial eyes and ears, mended spinal columns, and the remaking of all our organs — including the brain. Today, two major trends are remaking surgery: transplantation and non-invasive procedures.

Trend #1: Transplantation

Transplantation had its origin during World War II. Severe burns prompted efforts to provide skin grafts, most of which were rejected by then-unknown immune processes. Several Nobel prizes later, skin grafting and organ transplantation became realities because the host-donor interactions became known. Kidney transplants were started in Boston in the 1950s, livers in Pittsburgh in 1963, pancreas in Minneapolis in 1966, and heart in South Africa in 1967.

At my parent institution, the Stanford Medical Center, our one-year survival rate for heart transplantation was originally 20 percent. Today, that rate is over 80 percent — a fantastic record when you realize that heart transplant patients are extremely ill people who would not have lived a month without this gift.

Worldwide, over 30,000 heart transplantations have been performed — today, so many transplantation operations of all kinds are performed that they are considered "old hat" for those doing the surgery. For the patient, transplantation approaches the miraculous as they receive what is essentially a new life.

One of the major barriers to transplant surgery is the lack of availability of transplantable organs. In California, we have the option of affixing a sticker on our driver's license informing the world of our commitment to being a donor. I hope this practice is widespread because it is extremely important to expand our organ banks. Another barrier to transplantation is cost. Any organ transfer costs many tens or hundreds of thousands of dollars. And the costs are not confined to the surgery alone, because after surgery ongoing intense surveillance is needed to be sure that rejection is not occurring.

Because of the scarcity of organs and high cost of the procedure, organ transplantation is age-rationed. Every medical center has its own protocols governing the upper age at which transplantation may be considered. I am fiercely against age rationing for almost everything, but transplantation is an exception to this rule. If I was presented with two patients of similar capacity and problems, one 30 years old and the other 90, and each needed a liver but only one was available, I would certainly choose the 30-year-old.

The research frontier is bursting with new projections of made-to-order organs. Just how the hazards and expense of this new capacity for renewal interfaces with our increasing needs as we age is anyone's guess. The possible scenarios become wild. Imagine if, at age 90, I'd like a new lung, two knees, an eye or two, and a new neck, and these are all available at the supply store with easy to install instructions, but they cost $6 million — and my credit card is maxed out already! There are no books to consult on how we will handle these new situations. The future will bring dilemmas that we can only dream of now. Our judgement and competence are going to have to mature at least as quickly as the high-tech companies produce new miracles.

Trend #2: Non-invasive surgery

Surgeons are acutely aware of the high costs of their craft. They have sought to lower the bills by various strategies. In 1992, Mayo Clinic doctors kept their patients in the hospital for 8.1 days after opening up a clogged carotid artery. In 1993, the stay dropped to 6.8 days and to 4.6 in 1995. I am sure it is less now — perhaps someday it will be on an outpatient basis, which would have been unthinkable several years ago. But these days, the unthinkable is becoming commonplace.

A major breakthrough that has enabled hospital stays to be reduced is known as "band-aid," or non-invasive, surgery. Surgeons have developed a way of accomplishing their tasks by using a tube inserted into the body. This removes the need to open a large area of the body with a long incision. Tubes are inserted via a natural opening, when such an opening is available, or by a small incision allowing passage of the operating tube, when a natural opening isn't available. For several decades, urologists and gynecologists used tubes to look into the urinary and reproductive organs. If the prostate became enlarged, or there was a tumor of the uterus, it could be removed through the tube. This ability has now been extended to most other parts of the body, chest, belly, and joints. Today, most appendices and gallbladders are removed via a tube. Even heart artery bypass surgery is being performed this way. If you can avoid a major surgical incision, you will save yourself discomfort, time, and cost.

The surgeon's ability to pursue these new frontiers has been greatly expanded by spectacular new capacities with x-ray machines. New scanners allow us to see remote tissues almost as though we were holding them directly in our hands. Surgeons are able, using new optical techniques, to do surgery several feet away from the patient, being intimately guided by image-enlarging lenses. Surgeons can perform procedures in other countries now, through telesurgery. Microsurgery has immense applications, enabling precisions never earlier guessed at. All of these things mean that the modern surgeon is as much an engineer as a physician.

A further benefit of virtual surgery is the ability to train young surgeons on simulated computer patients. Instead of the very uncertain apprenticing of surgeons-in-training in actual care of ill persons, young surgeons can have "flight training" and documented abilities before trying their skill on a real-life patient. This should give comfort to us all.

Knowing When to Say "Yes" to Surgery

As an internist, part of my job description is to keep my patients away from the surgeon. Internal medicine and surgery can be thought of as an adversarial relationship, in which the patient benefits from different approaches, all offered by concerned specialists. The internist seeks conservative, tentative solutions. The surgeon is more aggressive and tends to be more categorical in approach. Surgeons don't tolerate gray areas as well as internists. In the best-case scenario, a specific diagnosis is made, the correct solution is planned, and the solution is carried out, surgically or medically. Hopefully, surgery need not be carried out on an emergency basis, but can be performed instead with deliberation and full preparation.

My internist's conservatism about surgery doesn't always hold. I took zero time to overcome any hesitation when I diagnosed our daughter's middle-of-the night acute gallbladder attack. Her gallbladder was in the surgeon's pan within two hours. That is how the system should work.

Indications for surgery

Most indications for surgery are clear-cut. There is no need for debate in the case of tumors, major bleeding, certain injuries, and some infections. Hopefully, the surgery can be curative. Sometimes, however, operations are needed just to make a diagnosis. New technology is changing traditional surgical situations and finding non-surgical solutions. For example, leakage or rupture of an aneurysm in the abdomen used to require emergency surgery. Now there are new procedures under trial to approach this drama non-surgically. Even with cancers, there are now alternative treatments to major surgery. Breast and prostate come most notably to mind.

As an internist, I feel that making the correct diagnosis is the most important step in the surgical encounter. An operating table is no place for surprises, so it's crucial to have the diagnosis established with greatest clarity before the surgeon acts. Any qualified physician can perform diagnosis, but the best is your primary care doctor, because of his/her familiarity with all aspects of your life and medical condition. The history, physical examination, x-rays, and laboratory tests will be used to diagnose your condition. All treatment options — both medical and surgical — should be fully explored before any decision is made. This may take several doctor visits and further tests.

Don't be afraid to get a second opinion if there seems to be any doubt about the appropriateness of surgery. Patients are often embarrassed and uncomfortable about asking for another opinion for fear of ruffling the physician's feathers. Any good physician should welcome a second opinion. A patient's confidence is critical to any successful outcome, and having as much information as possible is just plain good medical practice.

A person facing surgery should learn as much as they can about the proposed procedure. The Internet's numerous health sites cover just about every topic about surgery that you can imagine. These sources will help you frame the important questions you will want to ask your surgeon.

Making sure surgery is necessary

If you're going to have surgery, you have to have faith that surgery is science, and ruled by rational practice. Unfortunately, studies have proven otherwise. Similar communities such as Boston and New Haven have different numbers of operations per hospital admissions for the same surgical procedures: hysterectomy rates vary from 20 to 70 percent; prostate surgery rates vary 15 to 60 percent; and tonsillectomy rates vary 8 to 70 percent. In 1930, one-quarter of all operations in the United States were tonsillectomies (I had one). The current general consensus, however, is that the operation is almost worthless. The number of back operations in a community corresponds directly with the number of doctors who do back surgery. Even the surgical rates for something as straightforward as appendicitis have been found to vary threefold between communities.

Because it is impossible to believe that disease occurs so much more in one community than another, we have to conclude the different rates result from the surgeon and the practice habits. These differences are frankly very embarrassing to the idea that surgery is science, and not habit-based. Strenuous efforts are underway to address these disparities. Maybe in some communities not enough operations are being performed, but it seems that we should be more worried about limiting than encouraging surgery.

Practice guidelines, a set of agreed upon standards, will hopefully even out surgery rates. We must make sure that it is not the supply of doctors that rule the number of surgeries, but the patients' needs. Hopefully, the new practice guidelines will lead to a more rigorous match of need and performance.

Surgery is the last — not the first — recourse.

When Surgery is Necessary:
Shopping for a Surgeon

Most referrals to a surgeon will come from your primary care doctor. It's important that your physician have worked before with the surgeon through many previous experiences, and that you feel assured that the two communicate easily.

The personal attributes of a surgeon should be the same as any physician:

- ✔ Available
- ✔ Affable

 ✔ Able

 ✔ Accountable

For a surgeon, I would also add the quality of strength. Surgery is a tough business. The ability to stand up to the rigors of this high-stress, high-pressure life requires physical and emotional stamina.

Getting the most out of your surgeon

As you interview a prospective surgeon, you should ask about his or her training. You should find out what the surgeon's experience is with the operation you're considering. No one wants to ever be a guinea pig, and you should feel secure in the knowledge that the surgeon has performed several hundreds of these operations. The next question should be the results of these surgeries. The surgeon is honor bound to be fully disclosing about his/her experience. You should check to be sure that your prospective surgeon is board certified. Before becoming a surgeon, a young doctor typically goes through four to seven years of further training after medical school. During this period, the fledgling surgeon assumes progressively greater responsibility and autonomy. At the end of the training, the about-to-hatch surgeon undergoes an examination, and, upon completion, is granted official certification by the American Board of Surgery — hence the term "board certified." This credential is virtually mandatory for a surgeon to gain acceptance to hospital and clinic appointment. Your confidence in the surgeon will be bolstered too by knowing the professional associations he/she maintains are of the highest standards. The hospital where the surgery is to be conducted is crucial too, because the operation itself is only a small part of the total experience, and you should investigate the quality of the post-operative care you may expect. Before you commit to a surgeon or having surgery performed on you, ask the surgeon the following questions:

 ✔ **Where did you graduate from medical school?** Schools in the United States and Europe are better.

 ✔ **Where did you receive your surgical training?** Major medical academic centers are better.

 ✔ **Are you board certified?** Almost mandatory.

 ✔ **How many of these operations have you performed?** Don't be the first, or the tenth. The more the better.

 ✔ **What are your results with this operation?** Expect candor but not perfection.

 ✔ **What are the potentials for side effects?** Honesty rules.

 ✔ **What professional associations are you affiliated with?** For example, the American College of Surgeons, American Medical Association, and County Medical Society are notable institutions.

What a surgeon should do for you

The surgeon should provide a detailed explanation, often with pictures, of the proposed procedure. The degree of discomfort and disability should be fully disclosed and predicted. How long and where recuperation will occur require other elements of preparation for surgery. You should also discuss what steps you can do to fortify yourself, nutritional issues, exercise questions, concerns about blood transfusions — everything should be laid out in advance. Every question should be asked and answered before entry to the hospital.

You want to make sure that your surgeon will be as interested in you after the surgery as before. One of my pet peeves is a surgeon who disappears after surgery, feeling that the job is finished. Health is never finished, and all the collaborators and guarantors of this health should stay involved until everything is resolved.

Most physicians welcome review and disclosure. The era of "reputation medicine" is being replaced by "results medicine." Just because a surgeon is a professor, has won many awards, and has a lot of diplomas on the wall does not qualify him/her to me. Much more important are the outcomes of the surgery. Deaths, complications, survivals, and so forth all lead to analysis. We all need to know who is good and who is not.

Having Surgery As an Older Patient

Age is rarely a disqualification for surgery. Old people need surgery too, and the older we become, the more likely there is a surgeon in our future.

One cause of surgery in older people is cancer. Cancer increases with age because cancer seems to result from a series of gene changes, each one of which depends on an earlier mutation to achieve the malignant status. The longer we live, the more risk of completing the mutation sequence, and the greater risk of a malignant tumor. On the other hand, cancer in old persons tends to grow more slowly as it develops.

A second heightened surgical risk for old persons is accidents. Old people fall down. Falls cause 10,000 deaths per year in old people. Motor vehicle accidents cause 4,000 deaths annually for older persons, and pedestrian deaths another 2,000 older people. Burns cause 1,000 accidental deaths per year in old persons. Older people must be vigilant against accidents. Some say that after all diseases are prevented or cured, accidents will always remain as the major cause of death for older people.

Other unique surgical considerations exist for older people. Preservation and improvement of function is a worthwhile goal of surgery. Prosthetic joints have helped hundreds of thousands of persons with disabling arthritis. Without question, artificial joints have been a huge advance, leading not only to longer lives, but also to lives of vastly improved quality. I have witnessed the broad smiles of hundreds of patients awakening from the anesthesia for joint replacement when they recognize that the pain that had been their constant companion has disappeared.

Special risks and considerations for older people

Certainly, older people face greater risks during and after surgery. Their reserves simply are not as great. Too much bed rest is particularly threatening to older persons. Pain relief in older people can be touchy too, because most pain medicines can lead to confusion — something that is never conducive to a smooth recovery from an operation.

The surgical team should work to have the older patient out of the bed as soon as possible after an operation, often the same day. Every effort should be made too to reestablish normal nutrition as soon as the clinical situation allows. The period of time following surgery is critical for good communication. Once again, your primary care physician should play a role in the postoperative period, even though he/she has been only a bystander to the surgery. Patients and families are always afraid of what they don't know, and the full and honest disclosure of the findings and results of the operation that your primary care physician can communicate to you helps to speed healing and confidence.

Yes, there is life after surgery

The older person should face the prospect of surgery with confidence, optimism, and courage. Surgery is a major stress — there is no way around it. But the stress is temporary and after it comes the prospect of survival, and of an improved life after the tumult has died down. Not all surgery is successful, however, and bad news does happen. The mature person can deal with life's downsides as well as the ups and accommodate whatever the surgery's outcome is. No situation is ever "hopeless." Although the medical world pretends to be able to predict accurately the future, we are still very much imperfect. Hope always remains, no matter what. Hope is an element of life, and as long as there is life there is hope. The word "hopeless" should not even be in the vocabulary of your surgeon, or any other member of your health-care team.

Part IV
The Part of Tens

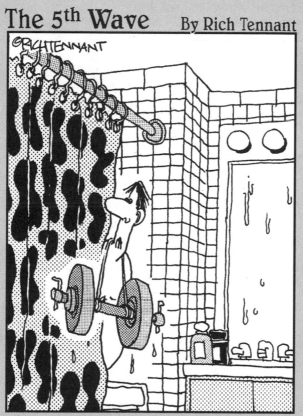

The 5th Wave   By Rich Tennant

"Okay, I know I need to start working out. Now, can I please have my soap-on-a-rope back?"

In this part . . .

Lists are great. They help keep you organized; they get right to the point; and they're fun and easy to read (Well, at least mine are!). I've put together five lists to get you on the right track to living longer.

Need the keys to a long life? Chapter 14 shows you what they are. Are you sitting down? Chapter 15 is designed to get you moving. Looking for the fountain of youth? Chapter 16 proves it may be through your stomach; look to this chapter for anti-aging diet tips. Losing brain power? Chapter 17 gives advice on how to keep your brain active. Taking medication? Chapter 18 gives you guidelines for taking medicine safely.

Chapter 14

Ten Keys to a Long, Healthy Life

• •

In This Chapter

▶ Knowing that how long and how well you will live is fundamentally up to you

▶ Staying active — both physically and mentally — can have a significant impact

▶ Realizing that the time is never too soon or too late to start — carpe diem!

• •

*O*h, if only you could simply find the fountain of youth and drink from it to stay young forever. Because no one has found it after thousands of years of searching, however, the time has come to face facts and take control of what you can in the aging process. This chapter presents ten tips to help you take charge of your own aging.

Creating Your Own Road Map to Life

Aging is a self-fulfilling prophecy. By creating your own road map to a long and healthy life, you establish the destination and the route. Without a plan, you are likely to be thrown off track when you encounter unexpected barriers along the way. Not only will your trip through life be shorter than it should be, but the scenery won't be as pleasant either.

You are in charge of your environment, so take charge. Life is to be lived actively, not passively. Routes are to be set, not accepted. Options are everywhere. Don't be a victim. This can be scary at times, but you can get through it. Courage and effective planning are the first keys to a long and healthy life.

Using It, Not Losing It

Most of your body is made up of tissues that allow you to move. Your muscles and bones are meant to be used. You need an exercise program — and not just on weekends, or when you're young, or when you go on vacation. Use your movement machinery every day. Remember the four forms of exercise:

- ✔ **Aerobics.** This kind of training improves your body's ability to move oxygen into every cell, where it helps to burn fuel.

- ✔ **Strength training.** An arm or a leg in a plaster cast quickly shrivels. The same goes for muscles and bones. They decay when you spend seven hours in front of the television or computer screen every day without exercising. Specific muscle-strengthening exercises are crucial if you wish to lift your great-grandchildren up some day.

- ✔ **Flexibility.** As you age, you run the risk of stiffening up. Keep your joints oiled up. Resist gravity's pull. As you age, your motto should be: Be an exclamation point, not a comma. Stay straight, not hunched over, by remaining strong and flexible.

- ✔ **Stay in balance.** Aging has a way of unsettling your internal compass. Keep it and your posture in a steady alignment by balance exercise.

For the young, exercise is an option. For the old, exercise is an imperative.

Eating Well to Live Well

Your car won't go very far if you feed it poor quality gasoline. Likewise, your body won't be able to hum and purr as you power through life if you put lousy fuel in your own tank. Favoring foods with too many calories — and the wrong kinds of calories — is easy. To live well, eat well by staying away from empty calories and processed foods. Eating a well-balanced variety of foods will help you in the long run.

Getting Enough Rest

The third part of your healthy body triad (after diet and exercise) is sufficient rest. The "everything in a hurry" lifestyle cuts our rest time too short. The treadmill of life seems to go faster and faster, allowing less opportunity for rest and recreation. Lack of rest results in stress, and stress is an active partner in many disease states. Don't rely on your physician to prescribe medicines to relieve stress, tension, and insomnia. You are your own best pharmacist for these problems. Give your body and mind an opportunity for respite.

Getting Involved

Using it and not losing it applies to the mind and spirit as well as the body. Stay actively involved in your environment and watch yourself for any tendency to disengage. No pill can replace the stimulus of remaining engaged with family, community, nation, and world.

Age should not determine when you retire. Work has major health benefits. You should retire only if you have some replacement activity that will provide similar stimulation and opportunity for continued growth.

Several surveys indicate that people who remain engaged live longer. And the more intimate the engagement is, the more powerful its life-extending potentials — and that includes sex. Don't worry about the negative stereotyping about sexuality and aging. Sex and its pleasures are not confined to the young. The physical problems of aging that affect sexual function are falling away with new medications and therapies for both men and women.

Staying Optimistic

A "can do" attitude will help you live a long, healthful life. Optimism breeds good results. Pessimism leads to negative outcomes. Optimism brings you energy to make the world a better place. Pessimism provides no opportunity for improvement. You can choose to see the glass half empty or half full. By seeing the glass half full, you will live longer.

Finding Meaning in Life

Because everyone is unique, you need to decide what a meaningful life is for you. Finding meaning in life is a highly personal affair. Meaning is not conferred, delivered, or inherited. I can't give you the answer, nor can your family members, your partner, your pastor, or your boss. A meaningful life for one person is not meaningful for another — you must create it out of personal experience. How meaningful is your life to you?

Staying in Control

The person most responsible for the extent and content of your life is not your parents, teachers, bosses, physicians, clergy, or Social Security administrators. You are in control of your own destiny. You can own and design your own life through an active process.

How well you take charge of your life determines your success. True, you must accept life's changes. Bills come due all along life's trajectory, and you can't keep charging the account to another payer. You created the bill. You must pay for it. No one wishes to be broke, and the soundest strategy to staying strong is to maintain control. Don't hide, don't depend, don't delegate. Do the work yourself and stay solvent. By controlling your life, you will gain a quiet self-confidence that gives you strength to change what should be changed and to accept what must be accepted.

Embracing Responsibility

Everyone talks about the "right to die." But what about the "responsibility to live"? Responsibility means maintaining an active search for a larger meaning for one's life. For most, this involves a repayment to the world around us for the privilege of the wonder of being alive.

The art of being responsible varies from person to person. For one person it means helping grandkids with their projects, for another it means environmental volunteering. For one person it means staying healthy through exercise and good diet, for another it means being a foster parent for someone less fortunate. There is still an awful lot of important and needy work to be done in this world, and age is never an excuse for turning your back on it.

Responsibility depends on knowledge. An animal or a newborn knows no responsibility, but the more we learn and experience, the greater our responsibility becomes. Older people have more responsibility because they have affected the world through their actions during their long lives. Entering my eighth decade, I welcome the burden of increased responsibility. I like to think I can handle it more equitably and capably than at younger ages. My rights endure, but my responsibility grows. That feels good.

We cannot assert our rights without accepting responsibility. Older people need to be a resource to our communities and nation — not a liability. Encouragement and embrace of responsibility will enrich us all.

Accepting Aging as a Normal Part of Life

Aging is not a disease to be cured, but a normal phase of existence. Understanding this concept changes everything we think about aging, including how we work with our physicians. Physicians should assume the role of teacher and health advisor. Physicians should cure sometimes, ease often, and comfort always. When you're older, chronic ailments become the predominant problems, and a different mind-set and therapeutic approach are appropriate. Your physician should be able to alleviate symptoms and preserve function. Having a good physician helps, but your best doctor lives within.

Chapter 15

Ten Reasons to Get Moving

As Chapters 1–13 indicate, I am a huge advocate for exercise. In fact, those chapters give you at least 20 to 30 reasons to exercise. The real challenge would be to find any reasons (aside from injury or serious illness) *not* to exercise!

Writing the Master Prescription

Exercise is more powerful, more dependable, safer, cheaper, and more effective than any drug. No prescription can come anywhere close to being able to make these claims. Exercise comes awfully close to being the cure-all — the magic elixir — that mankind has sought for thousands of years. Certainly there are many effective and important medications, but if only the United States took its dose of exercise more regularly, we could substantially cut our multibillion- dollar drug bill.

Two factors conspire against exercise. First is a bias toward inactivity. Each generation moves less and less as the world becomes more mechanized. Physical activity is devalued. People ask, "Why walk when you can ride? Why stand when you can sit?" But your bones, muscles, and arteries need to move. Nothing can substitute for this fact.

Second is physicians' indifference. We doctors place little emphasis on exercise as the universal therapy in prevention. I had no classes about exercise in medical school and few medical textbooks devote chapters to exercise. Whether or not your doctor encourages you, however, exercise!

Keeping Cash in the Bank

The time is never too early or too late to start exercising. The older you become, the more essential movement becomes to your health. In youth, your body holds an abundance of reserve energy stored up to serve your needs. With the passage of decades, this energy diminishes. If you're inactive, your energy will diminish even faster. Exercise for the young is an option. Exercise for the old is an imperative.

Physical fitness is like cash in the bank. With a big balance on your statement you can be a big spender, but when the reserves are low you must watch how big a check you write. Exercise is cash. Hoard the habit. Exercise early in life and late in life. Most importantly, keep exercising late in life, and you won't go broke.

Breathing Easier

Your life is like a candle. Without oxygen, life is extinguished very quickly. Exercise improves your body's ability to move oxygen. During exercise, your body moves up to ten times as much oxygen as at rest. Exercise conditions all parts of the body's respiratory system to work more efficiently — including your heart, lungs, brain, muscles, and bones. A fit person of 70 has the same oxygen-moving ability as an unfit person of 40. To make yourself an efficient oxygen-moving machine, exercise.

Making Yourself Strong

The world's stereotype of older people is "old and weak," but what if we could change that to "old and strong"? I'll let you in on a secret: Growing weaker is not a part of aging. People get weak as they age because they don't work out. You can stay strong throughout your life by doing muscle-building exercises. That means weight training (also known as resistance exercises) in which you move your arms, legs, and back with some load applied to them. You can use exercise machines (available in all health clubs) or simple "free weights" such as barbells. Hey, cans of food can even serve as weights — anything that makes the muscles exert themselves. I've seen 90-year-olds living in nursing homes restore their withered muscles by pumping iron. If they can do it, you can too.

Staying Loose

Growing older should not mean feeling tied up in knots — muscle knots, that is. As you age, you tend to lose flexibility due to changes in the elastic tissues of the body. As you tighten up, you might find yourself crawling out of bed in the morning without your usual spring, or taking the elevator instead of the stairs.

Stretching exercises can help put the spring back in your step. You can keep your ligaments, tendons, and muscles loose by a regular program of stretches for every moving part of the body — from your neck to your toes. Stretching need not be vigorous or hurtful, and you can easily combine it with the muscle strengthening and balance parts of your exercise protocol.

Getting Balanced

Almost half of older people fall at least once a year. The result of such a fall can be broken bones — a substantial health hazard that causes a decline in your quality of life. You can prevent falls by wearing sturdy shoes with good grips, taking care that your rugs can't slip, and working on your balance. Tai chi and yoga are excellent ways to maintain your balance. Other simple balance exercises, such as the flamingo stand, have been shown to prevent tendency to fall. Falls are an increasing threat to your well being as you grow older. Minimize falls by exercising your balance skills.

Avoiding "Oh, My Aching Back!"

Thirty-one little bones actually make up your "back bone." Together, all these little joints can conspire to cause an awful lot of misery. Back pain is one of the main reasons for doctor visits and work absenteeism.

The best solution to back problems? You guessed it — exercise. By keeping the major torso muscles tight (that includes the tummy muscles as well as the back muscles) the back retains stability and doesn't chatter, rattle, or hurt.

Strong backs don't hurt. Weak backs invite distress. Failure to keep your back strong sets up a vicious cycle of pain/inactivity/weakness/pain. Keep your back strong as you age.

Hurting from Arthritis? Exercise!

Joints are subject to inflammation or arthritis. When irritated and arthritic, joints become stiff and painful. Because joints are located at the intersection of two bones, you must keep the bones' alignment snug. Muscles, ligaments, and tendons that surround the joint shouldn't be allowed to grow slack, saggy, and loose. A tent pole with loose cables will start to sway dangerously. So too will joints. While the common advice for arthritis used to be rest, now we know the answer is exercise.

The most common health complaint of older persons concerns arthritis. Maintaining a good exercise program should retard its development, and may even reverse some of its achiness after you encounter it.

Keeping a Healthy Mind

Depression is a dark spot in life that puts lots of good things into shadow. The many losses that come with growing older create a fertile setting for depression.

Antidepressant medications can be very valuable, but exercise is a simpler, cheaper, safer, and often as effective remedy. Many psychiatrists prescribe walking, swimming, or jogging for the blues. Exercise releases endorphins, which are the brain's "feel good" compounds. I suggest you put more endorphins into your life and help battle depression with exercise.

Knowing the Simple Basics

How hard? How often? How long? Simple questions, yes, but they can give you no simple, single, or sure answers. A few things, however, do apply to everyone. Like everything else, too much of a good thing can become bad. For every one person who overdoes exercise, however, one thousand under-do, hence the encouragement to "push exercise."

Everyone should do some exercises on five or six days of the week. A rest day is wise, even for someone in active training for competition. Exercise should be of such intensity that you sweat, but not so hard that you can't carry on a conversation. Exercise should be hard enough that you would rate it as a "7" on a scale of one to 10, with "10" representing all-out effort. Exercise should last at least 30 minutes each day. Exercise periods don't need to be continuous and can be accumulated during the day by spaced out efforts.

You need to find an exercise program that fits you. Exercise is not something to be added on to your life — exercise must fit into your life. You must be comfortable with the whole proposition. I give this solemn promise: The more physically active you are, the healthier and happier you will be for the rest of your days.

Chapter 16

Ten Best Anti-Aging Diet Tips

In This Chapter

▶ Knowing the right foods to eat

▶ Remembering your vitamins and minerals

▶ Watching your fluids

*N*othing comes and goes faster than the latest fad diet. The basics of a healthy diet, however, have always remained standard. This chapter presents ten diet tips that will help keep you fit for life.

Getting a Perspective on Carbomania

What's best, a high carb, low carb, or no carb diet? Plenty of best selling books explore the answers. Unfortunately, most of the latest hot diet books are wrong and following some of those diets can be dangerous.

The only way to balance a pyramid is on a broad base. Any ancient Egyptian could've told you that. The same rule applies to the familiar Food Pyramid. The Food Pyramid has carbohydrates, including vegetables, grains, and fruits, as its foundation. Fifty to sixty percent of the day's calories should come from carbohydrates.

Carbohydrates are the bulk of the diet of most people on the planet. You could say that the world runs on carbohydrates. Not only do carbohydrates give you energy, but carbohydrate-rich foodstuffs also serve as a source of other good things such as vitamins, fiber, and minerals. Carbohydrates are nature's best foods. The exception is pure refined sugar, which contains no nutrients. Unfortunately, our natural sweet tooth has become unhealthfully hooked on sugar. People in the United States, in particular, consume too much sugar in soft drinks, pastries, frosted cereals, and the like.

When it comes to carbohydrates, don't be simple — be complex. Seek the bulk of your day's calories from complex carbohydrates such as veggies, cereals, breads, and fruit. These carbohydrates pay extra dividends with every mouthful.

Watching Fat Intake

Fat tastes good. Maybe that's because when our species had to fight to find enough food in the early days of our evolution, eating a lot of fat made sense since it contains the most calories of the three major food-stuffs. Now the pendulum has swung the other direction, and people today have too many calories available to them. Too much fat today means obesity and a higher production of cholesterol.

Obesity, diabetes, and clogged arteries are the predictable byproduct of a high-fat diet. The average diet of a person in the United States derives 37 percent of its calories from fat. A well-balanced diet should contain 30 percent or less.

As important as the total amount of fat in the diet is its source. Fats found in meats and dairy products raise your cholesterol. Fats from plants sources, such as olive oil, lower your cholesterol, and are some-times referred to as "good fats." The Food Pyramid advisory is 20 to 30 percent of calories from fat. Of that fat, only 10 percent should come from animal sources. Use lean meats, poultry, and fish. Remove visible fat. Don't fry. Use low-fat milk and cheese. Avoid animal fat whenever possible.

Being Pro-protein

Most of your body's structure is protein, and the only foodstuff that can provide your body with protein is protein. Although carbohydrate and fat are mostly interchangeable, there is simply no substitute for protein.

Meat is the usual source of protein calories, but vegetables contain amino acids (the building blocks of protein) too, some more than others. Soy is a particularly good vegetarian source of protein.

Older people need to maintain an ample protein intake because we tend to lose muscle with age. Too many older people fail to heed this advice because protein foods tend to be more expensive, require good teeth, and are harder to prepare. Lean meat, skim milk, and soy prod-ucts are particularly good protein sources as we age.

The downside of protein is not protein itself, but the fact that meat, particularly choice meat, has a high fat content. By eating chicken, fish, trimmed red meats, and soy products, you can obtain sufficient protein while keeping your fat intake low.

Roughing It

The food industry loves to refine and process foods, but in doing so one item is removed — fiber. How ridiculous it is to see drug store shelves stocked with all sorts of containerized fiber products when fiber is the structure of most natural foods! Primitive people didn't need to buy fiber. They ate it in large volumes — about ten times as much as we do. Low dietary fiber content may contribute to many medical conditions, from diverticulosis, to high cholesterol and colon cancer.

Raw fruits and vegetables are the prime sources of dietary fiber. Don't forget prunes — they deserve their reputation as digestive aids. If in doubt, seek out bran-containing cereals and breads to guarantee your fiber adequacy. Fiber has no calories and is terrific for relieving constipation.

Knowing Your Vitamins

Vitamins are like light switches in your body. You need a certain number to light up your life. But taking ten times the needed number won't make your life any brighter. The only thing taking too many vitamins will do is make your urine more expensive! For many people, vitamin excesses have replaced vitamin deficiencies.

Older people are the exception to this rule. Many eat vitamin-poor foods because of dental, social, drug, and financial issues. For this reason, I am quick to suggest a cheap multivitamin tablet daily for any older patient when I have any concern about the vitamin adequacy of their diet. The vitamin alphabet (A, B, C, D, E, and K) needs to be in everyone's regular food plan. Let me repeat, however, that vitamin *pills* are not, nor ever will be, a substitute for a well-balanced, intelligently planned food program. Good nutrition comes from a farm and not the druggist.

Drinking Fluids

You could actually think of yourself as a bag of water and not be too far off target. You are at least 60 to 70 percent water, but I bet you don't pay much attention to that part of yourself. Your kidneys take care of it for you. These wonderful organs filter 40 gallons of blood each day, getting rid of waste materials and regulating the levels of important body minerals. Urine represents only a tiny fraction of the work the kidneys do, and they do it with amazing precision.

As you age, some of your kidneys' precision erodes, and you may be in danger of dehydration or super-hydration. Older people should take care to ask about the effect of medicines. Many serve to squeeze the kidneys and therefore actually cause more fluid loss than they provide. And a word about coffee: Coffee stimulates water excretion so that the threat of dehydration is increased. Go easy on coffee. As you age, you should start to pay attention to your fluid intake and outgo. You should not take for granted any longer that your water machinery is automatic. Drink enough, but not too much. Good old H two O is the place to start, but juices and other drinks count too. Go easy on the soft drinks, though. They are nutritionally poor — and expensive to boot!

Taking Minerals

Minerals are important for your body's diet and structure. Salt and calcium are two of the substantial list of minerals that matter.

Around the world, different countries vary enormously in the amount of salt their people consume. And guess what? Countries vary in the incidence of high blood pressure too. This is no mere coincidence, because salt acts like a blotter, causing fluid retention and elevated blood pressure. When the body is young and lean, the kidneys do an awesome job of regulating the salt content of your system. With aging and obesity, this capacity diminishes. Hypertension can result, so watch your salt intake.

Magazines are full of information about calcium. The reason for this is the epidemic of hip fractures resulting from osteoporosis, in which the bones are fragile as a byproduct of low calcium intake. One and a half grams of calcium per day (three glasses of milk's worth) should be in all our daily diets, particularly if you are a woman. If milk is not your favorite food, take a calcium supplement.

Supplementary iron, especially for pre-menopausal women, may become an issue since menstrual blood loss may provoke an unsuspected iron deficiency state. Once again, however, a good, well-balanced diet almost always covers the essential needs.

Consuming Alcohol

For thousands of years, humans have drunk alcohol. For some, alcohol is a pleasure, and for others, it is a curse.

The alcohol dilemma has become more complicated by the medical news that a moderate amount is good for your health. Two questions immediately come to mind. How much alcohol is moderate? And what about those millions of people for whom alcohol is a poison as murderous as cyanide?

For those for whom alcohol is a toxin, the bad news is that they can't (not *shouldn't*) drink. Their lives and the lives of their loved ones depend on their restraint. For the nontoxic alcohol consumers, moderation is somewhere between one drink per day for small people and two per day for big people. This definition is very crude, however, and must be individualized. As you age, the same considerations apply, although probably more so. Whatever you drink, do so within reason.

Eating Just the Right Amount

You should eat often and in small amounts. For millions of years, our ancestors ate wherever and whenever they could. Rations were sparse. They didn't have three well-balanced meals.

Today, all the food you could ever want is available whenever you want. This abundance has evolved into the common pattern of a cup of coffee and a bagel for breakfast, sandwich and a soft drink for lunch, and then a mountain of food for dinner. This gorging meal pattern leads to the twin burdens of obesity and high cholesterol levels.

People today eat too much and at the wrong times. Less fat and more meals are the best program for nutritional health. A low-fat, nibbling diet, plus lots of exercise, would go a long way to decreasing the numbers of people in the hospital. Think less and more — less calories and more snacks.

Spicing It up with Variety

Probably the most important of the anti-aging diet tips is variety. The best diet is a mixed one, which regularly represents all of the basic food groups. Most major nutritional scientists will back me on this.

Advertisements encourage one food product over another. Unfortunately, if you listen to this message, you won't get enough variety. Your grocery cart should contain many types of purchases, and the more without packaging, the better. Some preserving and processing are necessary, but remember that our digestive systems evolved without the benefit of the food industry. Diverse, unprocessed foods are better for our health than products in fancy wrappers offered by the food industry.

Chapter 17

Ten Ways to Use, Not Lose, Your Mind

- -

In This Chapter

▶ Keeping things — life, love, loss, and more — in perspective

▶ Challenging yourself to learn something new

▶ Staying connected with family, friends, your community — and yourself

- -

*Y*our brain needs to work out just the way your body does. With no action, your brain will become "flabby" and shrivel. With more action, the connections between your brain cells will multiply and the size of your brain will actually grow.

Working Your Brain as a Muscle

Like your biceps, your brain needs to be flexed to be robust. If you do an activity frequently, the part of the brain that is responsible for controlling that function grows larger. So if you are an accomplished typist and type daily, the part of the brain that deals with small motor skills will be larger, as more connections between brain cells are formed. Conversely, when part of your brain isn't used, the corresponding brain area shrivels up like a leg in a cast. By challenging yourself in a constant variety of activities, blood flow, oxygen, and nutrients are directed to various parts of the brain. You'll stay sharp and productive. The brain is your master computer. You need to keep clicking your mouse if you want your mind to be bright and lively.

Hitting the Road

Travel provides new experiences, which are great stimuli for the brain. Anyone who wants to stay young at heart should maintain a healthy curiosity about how things are done on the other side of the globe — or on the other side of town! Sure, they say getting there is half the fun, but the other half of the fun comes from being introduced to new ways of living. Experiencing how other people eat, drink, dress, work, play, and think gives you a broader perspective. You'll recognize that not everyone is just like you and your family, and maybe change or add to your own rituals. A traveled brain is a fuller brain.

Drawing from Your Experience and Wisdom

Some wise person once said, "Not all old people are wise, but all wise people are old." The opportunity to grow wise certainly is one of the advantages of being older. You may gain wisdom as an unintended (and precious) byproduct of extended experience. And it's true that you learn more as you go through life. Failure can be a particularly effective teacher, if you decide to try to learn something from the experience. Wisdom grows slowly as you gain tolerance and a sense of time and history, and you begin to accept that the world is essentially imperfect, but can be improved upon. With wisdom, you know that no situation is without hope and that time is a powerful healer. It is certainly true that aging usually brings with it a sense of loss. Wisdom allows a widened perspective into which the ups and downs can be more easily allocated.

Managing Stress and Keeping Cool

Stimulation is good for the brain, but too much stimulation is harmful. Stress bruises the brain and can cause scars. After prolonged exposure to hurtful stimuli, the structure of your brain actually changes. Time plays an important role, too. People seem to be resilient enough to withstand short bursts of stress, but when the stress keeps coming like successive high tides, their brains become overwhelmed. As the brain loses its capacity to react, damage results. Even the small worries, over time, can be damaging.

Everyone needs stress-busting techniques, whether it's keeping a sense of humor, getting a pet, or exercising. Growing older helps in busting stress. Older people, by their added decades of experience, become better equipped to sort out what is and what isn't worth fretting over. And it really does turn out, in the long run, that most everything is small stuff.

Getting older has a big emotional benefit: emotional highs and lows become less pronounced. Hurts hurt less and don't last as long. Clinical surveys show that anxiety, anger, and hostility occur more often in younger people than in older people. Of course, as you age, you still experience both tenderness and pain. However, added experience takes the sharp edges off. An "I've been there; I've seen that" attitude is a good buffer against situations that might have caused distress at an earlier stage in life.

The older brain surges less, but knows more.

Being a Life-Long Learner

Why stop learning when you get a high school or college diploma? Learning is a life-long affair. My goal has been to try to know everything about something, and something about everything. Numerous studies show that education helps you live not only better, but longer.

Age is no barrier to learning. In fact, the brain's capacity to create and manipulate ideas grows richer as you get older. And every day, new opportunities for life-long learning are popping up, as witnessed by the huge success of the Elderhostel program. (The Elderhostel program sponsors worldwide educational seminars usually held on university campuses during vacation times — and it's free.) Learn a language, learn how to play a musical instrument, be a docent, or start a vegetable garden. The Internet, too, is an educational tool that allows access to a vast encyclopedia of facts and ideas.

As you age, you should count your riches not by how much wealth is in your checking account, but how much knowledge is in your head. You're never too old to stop adding to this account.

Earning Your Good Citizen Stripes

No one is an island. The older you become, the greater your responsibility for the world in which you have lived. As you age, giving back through public service is a way of paying back what society has given you.

Get involved with your community. Not only does getting involved help your community, it helps you. When you age, withdrawing and becoming isolated is all too easy, particularly after the loss of a spouse. The world needs you, regardless of your age! And when you think about it, the world needs you more now than it needed you last year or ten years ago because you're more valuable now than you were then.

Seek ways to be a good citizen. Vote, go to town meetings, take classes, do environmental work, counsel, teach, write letters to the editor, express yourself, and be necessary. Don't wait to be drafted to be a good citizen — volunteer to be one!

Staying Creative

Novelty is the spice of life, but finding new outlets for learning over and over again takes energy. Sure, you may be tempted to choose the sofa over the high wire, the rocking chair over the ski slope or coral reef, but, like the turtle, you can't get anywhere if you don't stick you neck out a little bit.

As you age, your brain should take to new ideas and opportunities more easily because you have seen and learned more than when you were younger. But you need some creativity to spark action. You can experience creative moments in your later years as well as in early years, but doing so takes energy and some courage. Keep trying new things, even if you might fail. Failure is a much richer life credential than security and comfort. When you no longer have the opportunity to fail, you will.

Remaining creative does not necessarily mean performing heroic deeds or painting the next Mona Lisa, but you should challenge yourself to shape life's happenings in new and improved ways — even in local and personal ways. Keep building yourself and your community.

Being Sense-able

The senses are your windows to the world. They are the portholes through which you can glimpse the larger world outside. Your senses let fresh air into your life. If you allow your senses to get dull, you will live a diminished life.

Don't take your senses for granted. Sight, hearing, smell, taste, and feeling are so intimately involved with the quality of everyday life that it's easy to assume they will always be there to serve you. Unfortunately, this might not be the case. A whole range of forces conspire to make you less "sense-able" as you age. Medications, for example, are notable for their detrimental affects on your antennae. Be aware of medication's effects.

Your senses may also become damaged from injuries caused by bright light or loud noises. You might not notice this subtle damage for years at a time, but don't let this fool you into assuming your eyes and ears are invulnerable. Like the rest of you, your eyes and ears need to be protected from abuse.

Have your senses medically evaluated every so often to be sure that you are not missing an early sign of deterioration. Take care of your senses. You'd be in a bad way without them!

Fighting Alzheimer's Disease

Alzheimer's disease is a demon loose in the land. We need to fight to eliminate this disease and the threat it poses to older people. The possibility that Alzheimer's disease may blight all our good work spoils the whole effort of living lives of vitality, competence, and meaning.

I am optimistic that recent knowledge has put science on several hopeful paths to eliminating Alzheimer's disease. In the meantime, before that glorious day is at hand, several strategies are appropriate. First, help take care of the poor souls and the families of those who have the disease. Second, do all you personally can to avoid the disease yourself. One possible action is to continue learning because educated people show lessened or later evidences of Alzheimer's disease. Take estrogen if you are a woman. Consider taking an anti-inflammatory medication because early experiments show promise with these drugs. Finally, support the Alzheimer's Disease and Related Disease Association (ADRDA). Their strong efforts to encourage medical research are our best hope to wakening sooner rather than later to that grand morning when Alzheimer's disease will be history.

Revering Memory

Sure, your memory isn't what it used to be. What is? Time takes a toll on your mental capacity to recall. Registration, retention, and retrieval are the three stages of your memory bank. It is how you deposit and withdraw your experience. We know that older persons' brains cannot retrieve as many items than the brains of younger persons. With training, an older person can far outperform an untrained younger person when challenged with a memory test.

How your memory is used is just as important as how old you are in determining what you recall. Many drugs, alcohol, and some medical conditions (including depression) serve to diminish memory-storing capacity. Change what you can and accept what you must, but know the difference.

Put your memory back to work. Remember the names of your high school teachers and classmates. Recall you grandkids' birthdates. Write down the names of all the states, and those that you have visited. Keep depositing into your memory bank.

Chapter 18

Ten Guidelines for Taking Medications Safely

• •

In This Chapter

▶ Developing a partnership for safe medicating between physician, pharmacist, and patient

▶ Staying informed of the pros and cons of your medications

▶ Communicating when the results aren't what you expected

• •

*O*lder people need to be cautious when taking medication. Adverse drug reactions are at least 20 percent more common in older folks than younger. The ten tips in this chapter apply to all medications, from the simplest and safest to the most complex and hazardous. Medications can be extremely helpful in preventing unwanted medical conditions, but only if they're taken properly!

Trying to Simplify, Simplify, Simplify

Hundreds of times I have interviewed a new patient, and along the way I have asked them to empty their purse, pockets, or paper bags of their current medications. Six, eight, or ten vials tumble out. Patients get to a point where they take some medications just to treat the side effects of another medication! Often, taking fewer medications instead of more is better. And don't forget, good diet, exercise, and rest are strong medicines too, and they are cheap, safe, and easily available.

Knowing When to Stop Taking a Medicine

Never take a pill just because so-and-so once prescribed it — maybe for reasons that are no longer present. Don't keep taking a medicine just because you needed it once upon a time. Be aware of the expiration dates on your pill bottles — they are there for your protection. Finally, never, never take someone else's medicine.

Knowing When to Continue Taking a Medicine

Insulin, thyroid, and heart medications are good examples of medicines that require continued use. If you are tempted to stop taking a medication for some reason, check with your doctor first. Forgetfulness and cost are probably the main reasons why people fail to take their medicines, but minor side effects such as nausea or weakness might also prompt an interruption in dosage. Check with your doctor about changing the dose or even changing the medicine, because usually acceptable substitutes are available.

Taking the Lowest Dose Possible

People, especially older people, should always take the lowest possible dose of a medicine. Your physician should be aware of this, but is probably accustomed to prescribing a standard, higher dose for young people. Take responsibility by asking your doctor about a lower dosage.

Although you should take only the lowest amount necessary for benefit, you must also take however much you need to take to produce the desired effect. I have often increased the dose of an ineffective prescription to find it working at the correct and higher dose.

Updating Your Prescriptions

Check your prescriptions regularly to see whether the disease diagnosis for which a medication was originally prescribed is still appropriate. Medical conditions change regularly. When they change, your doctor should take a new look at your prescriptions.

Keeping Your Drug History Current

Always update your drug history. Note whether or not a medicine worked for some condition. Did the medicine cause a problem? An ongoing inventory of medication experience is important because the memory is a faulty device, so noting the facts when they occur is best. Because medication use is a complicated business, it makes terrific sense to create a personal drug diary that lists time and circumstance of unusual drug actions or inactions. For example, a drug may be more or less effective when taken with a meal, and you can be a handy detective in helping find out these discrepancies.

Staying Aware of Possible Drug Interactions

Although you might not have a problem with a medication when you take it alone, adding other medications to the mix can cause bad interactions. Whenever you start taking a new drug with a previous prescription, be extra cautious of unexpected side effects and contact your doctor immediately if they occur.

Medications are complicated enough when used singly, but combinations really increase the complexity. The personal drug diary that I mention in the previous section is a good way of keeping track of unexpected and unpleasant interactions. Many pharmacies now have computer systems that will track your prescriptions and identify any possible interactions. Although these can be very helpful tools, they're certainly no substitute for strong communication between you, your doctor, and your pharmacist.

Measuring Your Drug Levels

Ask your doctor about measuring the levels of the drugs in your blood stream. This technique is extremely helpful in deciding the proper dosage for you. For example, the "killing dose" of some antibiotics — the dosage needed to eliminate the bacteria — is no longer guesswork because your doctor can measure the drug's action on the bacteria.

Correction formulas are available that allow dosage adjustment when certain organ functions are impaired. For example, if your kidneys were found not to be excreting at normal rates, some drugs come in lower doses, tailored to the degree of the kidneys' impairment.

Taking Medications as Directed

I know, you hear this all the time, but not taking medicines properly is the biggest problem older people face. A medication is not going to be effective if it remains in the pill bottle. Sometimes older people take too much medication too often, but much more commonly, they don't take enough. Drug blood level assessments (which I discuss in the previous section) can help a physician clarify if a patient is taking too much or too little medication. Involving another person to assure that a medication is taken properly can work. Or simply counting how many pills remain in the bottle after a set period of time gives an indication of compliance.

Some medications need to be taken first thing in the morning, others on a full stomach, others when upright. The advisories differ, so be aware of these instructions as well as the usual "times per day" advise. If, after an appropriate interval of several days, the medicine is not working as your doctor predicted it would, call your doctor for further advice.

Minimizing the Number of Doses

Ask your physician about medications that can be taken in the simplest doses. Drug companies have found, not surprisingly, that the compliance of once-per-day dosing is much better than when a drug requires multiple daily doses. Consequently, they are developing more medications that can be effective in more simple doses.

Part V
Appendixes

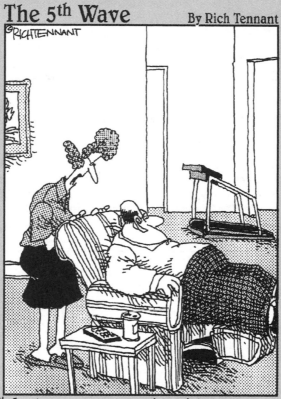

The 5th Wave — By Rich Tennant

"You know, anyone who wishes he had a remote control for his exercise equipment is missing the idea of exercise equipment."

In this part . . .

Located here are two quick references for important information on medication and common conditions and treatments. Appendix A offers a guide to medicines that you are most likely to encounter as you age. Appendix B provides tables on the most common ailments suffered by older people and methods used to treat them.

Appendix A

A Guide to Medicines

● ●

*W*hen it comes to medications, we've come a long way. One hundred years ago, less than 2 percent of what was being prescribed by physicians in the United States had any clinical value. In fact, a review of the first *Merck Manual* (still considered the ultimate source for all information on medications), is a slender 262 page booklet published in 1899. While this book was highly valued by the practitioners of the time, rereading of this material is frightening. Remedies and confidence placed in the prescriptions for the diseases of that time make you wonder how patients survived their treatment. Today, the *Merck Manual* is in its 18th edition and runs 2,600 pages. There is no better symbol for the explosion of knowledge and options when it comes to medication.

The number of prescriptions that doctors write is also ballooning, and older people are taking most of that medicine. Doctors write two billion prescriptions each year. That's eight for every man, woman, and child in the United States! Older people average 12 prescriptions per year. Many are unnecessary.

My professor of medicine in medical school taught us students in his first lecture, "Ladies and gentlemen, I have done much more good in the world by stopping medicine than by starting it." Writing a prescription saves the doctor time. Addressing behavior changes that may help your problem takes more time than prescribing a pill. Side effects are also an important consideration. Every medicine brings side effects, and the older the patient, the more likely the side effects will occur. Older people react differently to many drugs because their capacities to transport and excrete the drugs are different. For this reason, doctors should reduce the doses of most medicines for patients over 70 years of age.

How Drugs Work

Drugs work by altering the cellular signal settings so that the cause and effect of the disruption in biochemical service is reversed. Used properly, drugs enable healthy patterns to be established again. Of course, until now, none of this basic mechanism of drug action was understood. Medications were used simply because they were found — by chance — to bring down fever or ease achy joints. Quinine and aspirin became popular because they worked, not because we understood why they worked. Fortunately, pharmacological science is rapidly revealing how and why medications work at the cellular and genetic levels. The cause and effect linkage is understood better all the time. Someday, our specific understanding will allow us to custom-design remedies.

Voltaire observed, "Physicians' practices consist of prescribing medicines, of which they know little, to persons of whom they know less, for reasons of which they know nothing."

The effectiveness of medications has another component besides just the local action at and in the cell. By knowing the biochemistry of medications (how they fit into the receptor sites), the pharmaceutical industry can predict which shape of drug molecule is likely to have a desired effect on the cell. This is called *bio-availability* and implies that the drug compound is carried to the desired tissue site to perform its desired action, usually by the blood stream.

Bio-availability is a big part of what makes drugs work. Like an express package, a drug must be delivered to the right place in the right amount at the right time. If the drug doesn't reach its prospective destination, it can't work. If a pill behaves like a marble and goes through the intestinal tract without being absorbed, it can't work. If a medication for meningitis can't get from the blood across the brain blood barrier to treat the disease, it won't work.

Every primitive society had medications distributed through its apothecary, but the products were unproven and often dangerous. King Charles II of England, for example, died the victim of a horrible combination of "medications." In 1685, after suffering a stroke, he summoned his physician. The treatment began with substantial bloodletting. Then the doctor administered drugs — a series of laxatives, concoctions to induce vomiting, and enemas containing cinnamon, fennel, bitters, violets, and 15 other agents. A sneezing powder of hellebore root was prescribed. A plaster of pitch and pigeon dung was applied to the soles of his feet. Despite all this (or more likely *because* of all of this), his condition deteriorated. An emergency dose of 40 drops of extract of human skull was given. The sorry king died as a mixture of herbs, animal extracts, and ammonia was being forced down his throat.

Human beings are complex. Every person's case is different. The same drug does not work the same for every person. (The idea that one size fits all works much worse for drugs than it does for clothing!) Just because a new medicine has worked out on ten people doesn't mean it won't harm the eleventh person. Any wise physician won't be the first on the block to prescribe a new remedy — regardless of how much marketing hoopla accompanies its introduction.

New Drugs and Old Patients

Pregnant women and newborn babies get loads of special attention from drug companies. Products for these constituencies go through additional testing to ensure that their products have no adverse effects.

Unfortunately, people on the tail end of life span — older patients — go virtually unexamined. No particular effort goes into seeing whether a drug has any unintended negative effect when given to older persons. Why? The answer is simple: because of the expense of additional test-ing. Older people are even more heterogeneous than the population as a whole because they often have several medical conditions and are taking a variety of medications. Therefore, to corral a group of older persons and sort out the effects of the new medication is untidy and uncertain. As a result, extra caution is required when an older person tries a new drug. Every case is truly an experiment of one.

How Medicine Affects Older People Differently

Older people are different. Their body composition is different because as body water decreases with age, body fat goes up. When you consider that some drugs dissolve in water and others in fat, you can imagine that drugs will distribute themselves differently in an older person than in a younger one. A drug may be much more potent or much less potent as its bio-availability is changed in an older person's system.

Drugs tend to be excreted either by the kidneys or the liver. If an older person has any decline in functioning of the kidneys or liver, a drug may just keep going 'round and 'round in a circulation before being excreted, which increases its chance of toxicity.

Most oral drugs are absorbed in the small intestine, and because older people lose some of the absorptive surface in the intestine, medica-tions don't have as much of a chance to get into circulation. Also, because evidence suggests that cellular receptor sites may diminish with age, being certain of a drug's effectiveness is difficult.

Aging particularly changes the effectiveness of certain nervous system drugs. Some sedatives, such as phenobarbital, may become agitating. Other sedatives sedate too long.

A Brief Course in Common Drugs

Of all the thousands of drugs, older people only commonly use seven main categories. These are:

✔ **Blood thinners.** The most common type of blood thinner is coumadin, also called warfarin. This drug is used to keep the blood from clotting. Clotting is frequent in situations of prolonged bed rest or after surgery. Irregular heart beating (such as atrial fibrillation) also leads to clots. Coumadin is routinely monitored by blood tests to carefully track its action in a patient. The main side side effect — which is major — is hemorrhaging. Sadly, I have witnessed fatal bleeding into the head of two of my patients — cases that still haunt me. Coumadin is also dangerous because its potency fluctuates depending on other drugs in your system, and even some foods. If you take coumadin, you must always be super-alert about potential side effects.

✔ **Anti-cancer drugs.** Because cancer is an overproduction of cells, the drugs designed for its treatment work by blocking cell division. Unfortunately, the cancer cells are not the only ones affected by these medications — all cells are inhibited in their division. The bone marrow that makes blood cells is particularly vulnerable. Regular blood tests are necessary when taking any anti-cancer drug.

✔ **Anti-inflammatory medicines.** These compounds, including aspirin, are probably the most widely used class of medicine in older patients due to the high incidence of arthritis in an aging population. All of these drugs, with minor exceptions, carry the potential of irritating the lining of the stomach and intestine. The first evidence of this common side effect is often bleeding from the rectum. The anti-inflammatory medications also interact with drugs of other classes, so that no one should regard their use casually. Use the smallest dose that works, for as short a period as possible.

✔ **Antibiotics.** These drugs are widely used to combat infection in patients of all ages, and are far over-prescribed. Antibiotics can have side effects that could conceivably, although rarely, be fatal. Some antibiotics can be directly measured in the blood, which can guide therapy. Low doses and short usage are wise.

✔ **Cardiovascular drugs.** Hundreds of kinds of cardiovascular drugs address conditions from high blood pressure and high cholesterol to weak heart action and irregular heart beat. Most of these drugs have unwanted side effects. High blood pressure medications may cause low blood pressure, which could provoke a stroke. Digoxin, used often to control rapid heart beats, can provoke slow heart rate and a stroke. Diuretics, which work on the kidneys to rid the body of excess water as in heart, kidney, or liver failure, are renowned for their mischief.

Diuretics are used to help the kidneys get rid of extra fluid that may have accumulated from various causes. Congestive heart failure, in which the heart's pumping capacity is diminished, is one of the most common indications. But just like all medications, diuretics have side effects, such as excessive potassium loss, leading to profound weakness.

✔ **Central nervous system medications.** Depression, hostility, and insomnia are common conditions in older populations. If an older person is low, we have drugs to make the person high. If a person is agitated, we have drugs to provide tranquility. The trick always is not to overshoot the intended target, and thereby cause more problems than you had wished. Again, go for low doses over a short duration.

✔ **Hormones.** Although hormone preparations come in many different flavors — insulin, prednisone, and thyroid, to name a few — sex hormone replacement protocols are the ones most commonly used by older people. For us older fellows, testosterone is the issue. Many doctors prescribe testosterone to their older male patients in efforts to enhance flagging sexuality and vitality. I am very cautious in this regard, because testosterone stimulates the prostate in ways not easy to predict.

The female sex hormones of estrogen and progesterone are on a firmer medical footing, in my opinion. Their value in offsetting cardiovascular problems, osteoporosis, and Alzheimer's disease is documented. But their potential to increase the risk of cancer of the breast and uterus should temper their use.

Despite my general enthusiasm for the estrogen-progesterone protocol, I do not advocate those drugs for my wife, whose mother died of breast and ovarian cancer, and whose sister and niece have had breast cancer. Further, my wife is a confirmed long-distance runner, which is a good insurance against circulatory problems and osteoporosis.

Even given all these caveats, medicines are wonderful. Not only are we living longer because of medicines, we are living better. Late-life quality has been markedly improved in the last ten years, and much of the credit for this goes to the pharmaceutical industry and to the medical system that prescribes its products.

Drugs and the "Placebo Effect"

How do we know if a drug is working? We perform a clinical trial. Clinical trials should be done in a double-blind fashion. The term "double-blind" refers to a setup in which neither the tester (the investigating physician) or the testee (the patient) knows whether the compound being dispensed is the real experimental drug, or is an inert compound that looks and tastes like the drug, but contains no active ingredient — in other words, a "sugar pill."

After the trial is completed and the results tabulated, then researchers reveal which was the real drug and which was the sugar pill. If the real drug performed better than the sugar pill, then activity is demonstrated. This is considered a "positive result." But what if both the real drug and the sugar pill work? What if the sugar pill was not quite so good as the real drug, but patients taking each still shared some improvement? I'll let you in on a secret — this is the most common result in all drug studies. The mere act of taking a drug — and the empowerment of doing something about a condition — carries benefit. Researchers call this improvement the "placebo effect."

The cover story of the January 9, 2000, *New York Times Sunday Magazine* dealt with the placebo effect. The article reviews sham surgical procedures, such as actual incisions on the knee or chest, and compared these with arthroscopy or mammary artery ligation performed for coronary heart disease. The placebo surgery experiments reveal that merely having the patient believe he/she had a relieving procedure performed delivered as much measurable clinical benefit as the "real thing." Merely drilling holes in the skull of some patients with Parkinson's disease, was as effective as a hole drilling plus other supposed definitive surgery! Of course, it is impossible to do "double-blind" surgery, as clearly the surgeon knows what incision is real and what isn't, but the evaluators of the results can be blinded.

The proven reality of the placebo effect, even in surgical operations, is humbling to the medical purist. No longer can the doctor or the drug company take credit for all the cures and improvement in a disease condition. Many operations and medicines that have come into regular, unquestioned use, are now subjected to the reappraisal demanded by the placebo effect. Different estimates place the power of the placebo as 35 to 75 percent of the active intervention. Many drug studies have even shown that the results of the placebo turned out to be better than the "real drug."

The value of the placebo is not just in the brain. Doctors commonly see actual improvement in blood pressure, pulse rate, and blood values. A placebo study of bronchodilators in patients with asthma showed that belief alone led to some opening up of the breathing tubes. The placebo effect is not all in the imagination. Most of the millions of doses of antibiotics prescribed by many practitioners for viral infections are placebos as well.

Appendix B

Common Conditions and Treatments

● ●

*B*y definition, the centenarians are the survivors. They are the ones who have escaped the major illness challenges to which the non-survivors have succumbed. A remarkably high number of centenarians report no health problems whatsoever, but of those who volunteer concerns, arthritis is the most commonly listed condition, followed by decreases in sensory capacity (both sight and hearing). Heart disease, cancer, and stroke also inhabit the lives of centenarians, as they do the lives of their predecessors. The following three tables break down information on the five major causes of death, the most common chronic diseases of persons over 65, and common older person conditions.

Five Major Causes of Death

Condition	Symptoms	Medical Treatment	Self-Management
Heart disease	Chest pain, shortness of breath, irregular heartbeat, weakness, lightheadedness	Pain relief, oxygen, blood pressure control, surgery as last resort	Moderate exercise, stop smoking, watch diet and weight, reduce stress
Cancer	Unexplained weight loss, unexplained mass, weakness, unexplained bleeding, blockage of bowel or bladder	Surgery, radiation, chemotherapy	Be informed, ensure correct diagnosis, follow treatment vigorously
Stroke	Paralysis, speech difficulty, loss of consciousness, memory loss, numbness	Blood pressure control, blood thinners, aggressive physical therapy	Work hard with therapist, stay involved with life watch blood pressure

(continued)

Five Major Causes of Death *(continued)*

Condition	Symptoms	Medical Treatment	Self-Management
Emphysema	Shortness of breath, exhaustion, cough	Treat infection, bronchodilators, steroids, oxygen	Stop smoking!, stay strong, practice deep breathing
Dementia (usually Alzheimer's)	Loss of recent memory, disorientation, poor judgment, speech difficulty	First make correct diagnosis, as some forms of dementia have good treatments while others, Alzheimer's disease for example, do not have good treatment — YET	Simplify life, keep mental activity up, exercise, avoid stress

* List compiled from data from the National Center for Health Statistics

Most Common Chronic Diseases of Persons Over 65

Disease	Percentage
Arthritis	48.2%
Poor hearing	32.0%
Hypertension	59.8%
Heart	18.3%
Diabetes	11.0%

* List compiled from data from the National Center for Health Statistics

Common Older Person Conditions

Condition	Symptoms	Management
Alzheimer's	Recent memory loss, poor judgment	Simplify life, keep mentally alert, avoid stress
Arteriosclerosis	Chest pain, leg pain, dizziness	Don't smoke, reduce cholesterol, exercise, one baby aspirin per day
Arthritis	Joint pain, swelling, decreased motion	Rest when irritated, keep flexible

Condition	Symptoms	Management
Back pain	Acute or dull pain, may go into legs	Limit activity, ice, watch amount of pain medication carefully
High Blood Pressure	No symptoms: regular check-ups recommended	Control salt, reduce weight, exercise, watch stress
Bronchitis	Cough, phlegm, fever, wheezing	Avoid smoke, drink fluids, breathe moist air
Cataracts	Fuzzy, blurred vision, problems with glare	Increase light, surgery
Constipation	Difficult bowel passage, pain, bloating	Fluids, fiber, avoid self medicating, possible use of laxatives
Decreased hearing	Loss of high tone sensitivity, problems with discerning sounds when in crowds	Regular hearing tests, keep wax clear, looking at source of sound or speech markedly improves comprehension, consider hearing aid
Depression	Sadness, loss of sleep, weakness, loss of appetite	Exercise, social involvement, ask for professional help
Diabetes	May be none, change in weight, fatigue, excess urination, vision change	Weight loss, exercise, medical care, insulin or drugs
Falls	Pain, swelling	Splint injury, elevate, Tylenol for pain
Flu	Ache, fever, weakness	Fluids, Tylenol or aspirin, rest
Hemorrhoids	Enlarged veins at anus, bleeding	Keep clean, avoid constipation and straining, cold compresses
Incontinence	Leakage or urgency	Avoid stimulants, urinate at specific time intervals, strengthen pelvic muscles with exercise
Insomnia	Trouble getting to or staying asleep	Avoid caffeine, avoid naps, avoid pills
Osteoporosis	No symptoms, no pain	Calcium, estrogen for females, exercise, discretionary use of medications

(continued)

Common Older Person Conditions *(continued)*

Condition	Symptoms	Management
Pneumonia	Cough, phlegm, fever, chest pain	Liquids, fever medications, antibiotics under physician care
Prostate problems	Difficult urination	Suspect infection, use antispasmodic medication, surgery
Sexuality, male	Impotency	Medical exam and diagnosis, watch drug side effects, Viagra
Sexuality, female	Lack of desire, discomfort, lack of opportunity	Desire and discomfort can be addressed by hormonal steps (either pills or creams), opportunity problem is addressed by keeping husband alive and healthy

* Gerontologic Society

Index

Notes

Notes

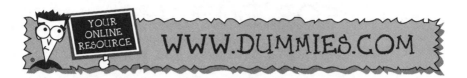
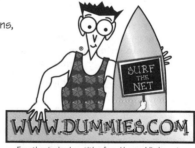
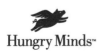

FOR DUMMIES
BOOK REGISTRATION

Register
This Book
and Win!

We want to hear from you!

Visit **dummies.com** to register this book and tell us how you liked it!

✔ Get entered in our monthly prize giveaway.

✔ Give us feedback about this book — tell us what you like best, what you like least, or maybe what you'd like to ask the author and us to change!

✔ Let us know any other *For Dummies* topics that interest you.

Your feedback helps us determine what books to publish, tells us what coverage to add as we revise our books, and lets us know whether we're meeting your needs as a *For Dummies* reader. You're our most valuable resource, and what you have to say is important to us!

Not on the Web yet? It's easy to get started with *Dummies 101: The Internet For Windows 98* or *The Internet For Dummies* at local retailers everywhere.

Or let us know what you think by sending us a letter at the following address:

For Dummies Book Registration
Dummies Press
10475 Crosspoint Blvd.
Indianapolis, IN 46256

™

**BESTSELLING
BOOK SERIES**